Karmic Regression Therapy and Karmic Reiki

Practitioner Manual

Part of

The One Therapy Home Experience

by **Martyn Pentecost**

**Originator of Karmic Reiki,
Karmic Regression Therapy and One Therapy**

First Published in Great Britain 2018 by mPowr (Publishing) Limited

www.mpowrpublishing.com
www.one-therapy.com

A catalogue record for this book is available from the British Library
ISBN – 978-1-907282-19-5

Book and Digital Design by Martyn Pentecost
mPowr Publishing 'Clumpy™' Logo by e-nimation.com
Clumpy™ and the Clumpy™ Logo are trademarks of mPowr Limited

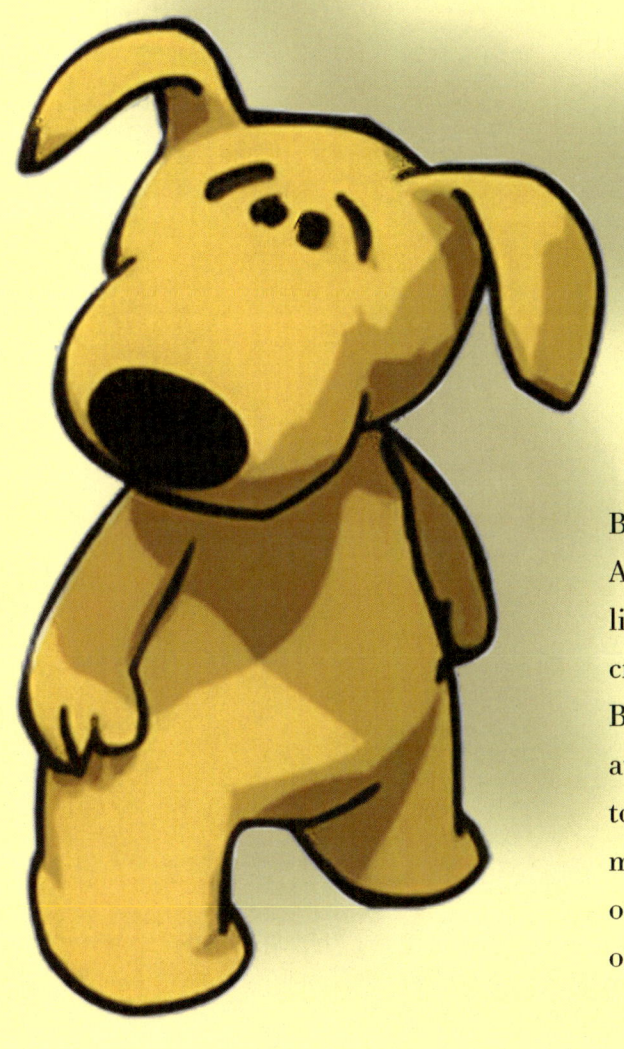

Made by Book Brownies!

Books published by mPowr Publishing are made by Book Brownies. A Book Brownie is about so high, with little green boots, a potato-like face and big brown eyes. These helpful little creatures tenderly create every book with kindness, care and a little bit of magic! Before shipping, a Book Brownie will jump into the pages—usually at the most gripping chapter or a part that pays particular attention to food—and stay with that book, always. This means that every mPowr Publishing book comes with added enchantment (and occasional chocolate smudges!) so that you get a warm, fuzzy feeling of love with the turn of every page!

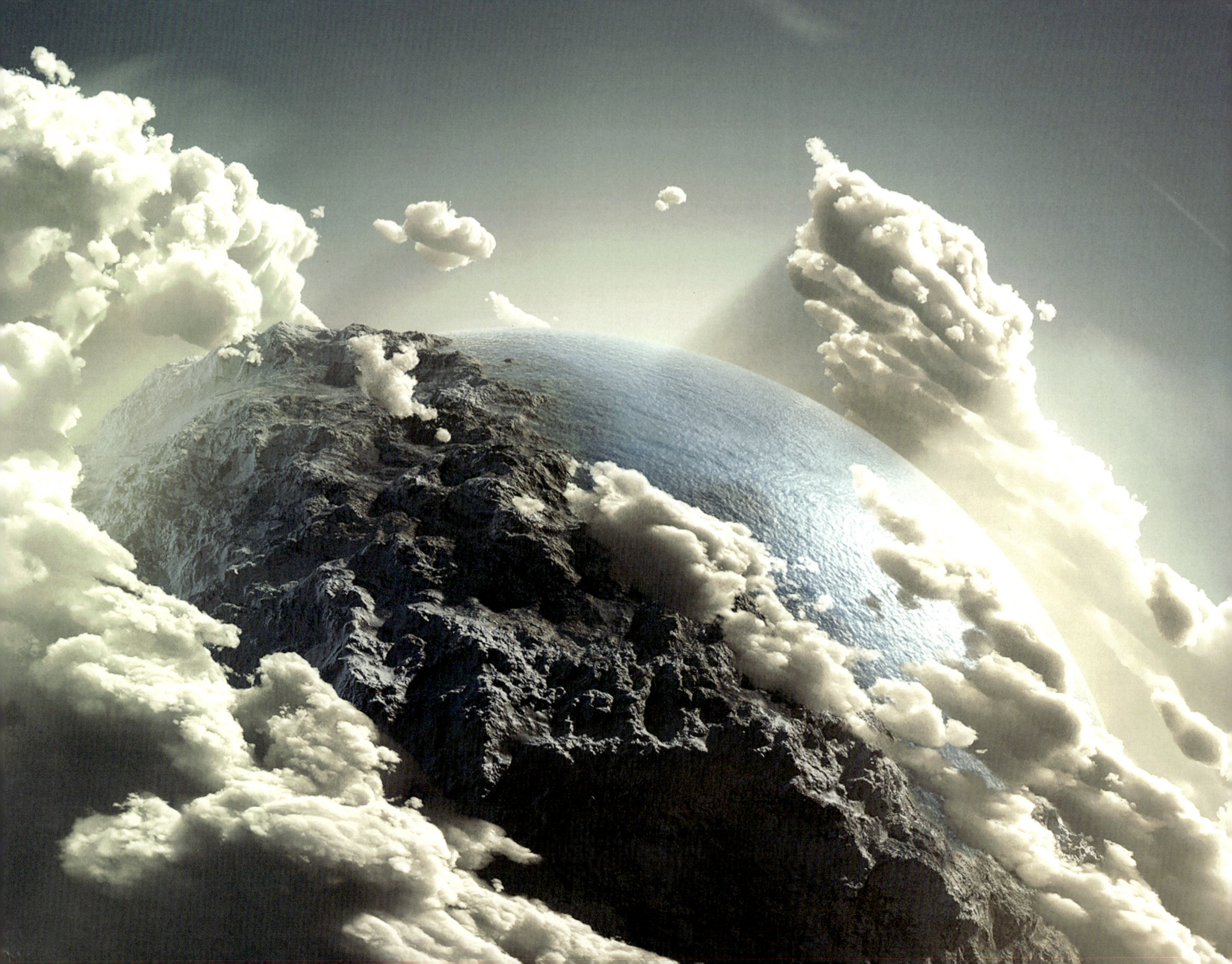

one

therapy home experience

celtic reiki realm & seer
vReiki & the reiki revolution
karmic regression therapy
psyQ
the viridian method

www.one-therapy.com

contents

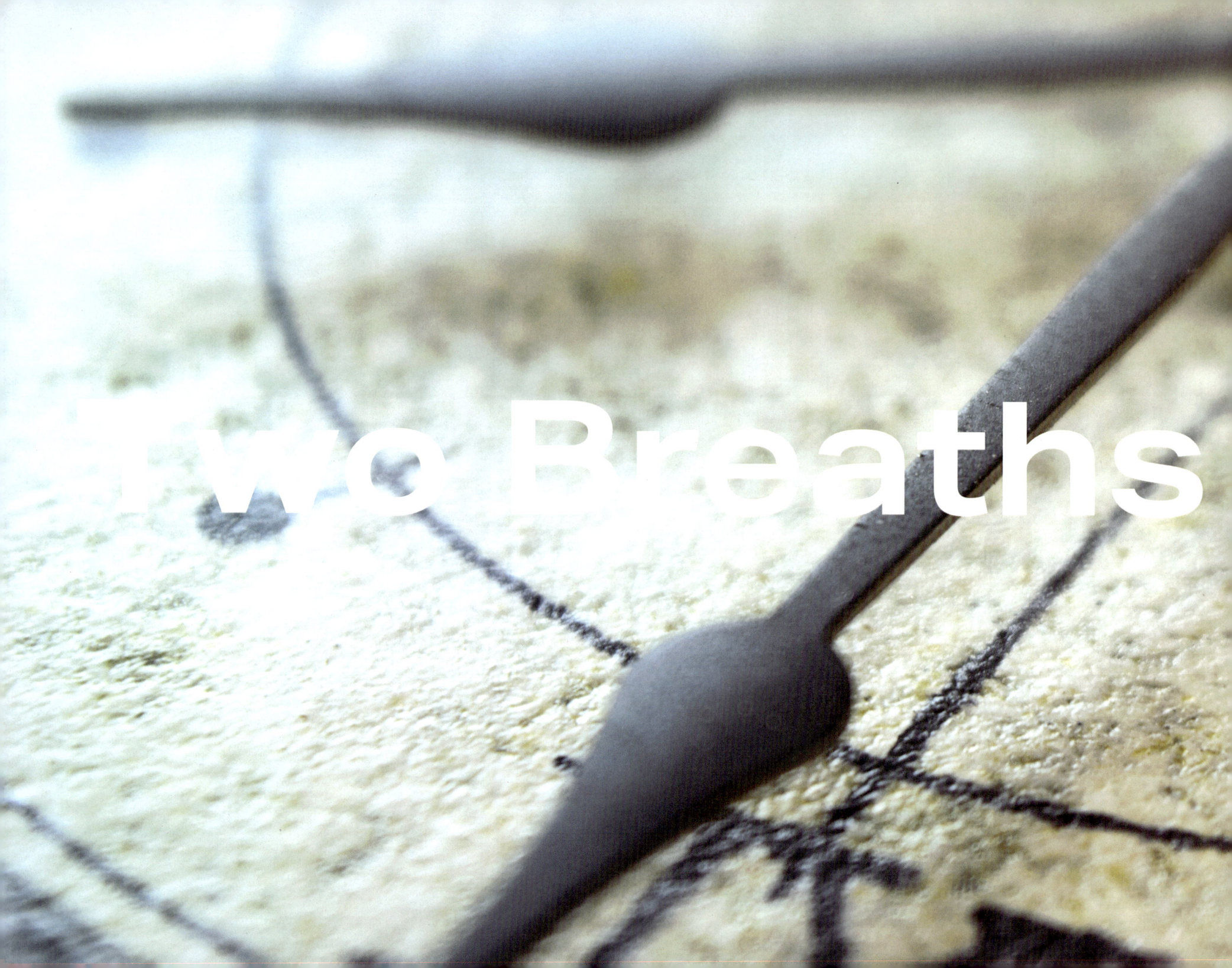

Two Breaths

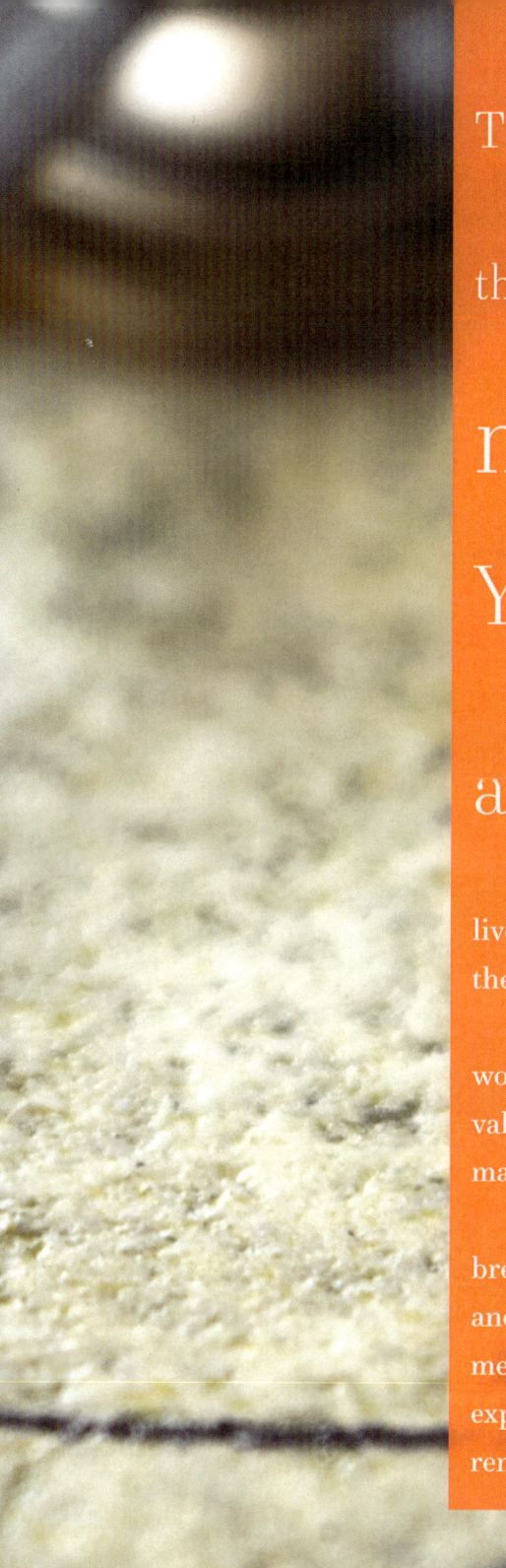
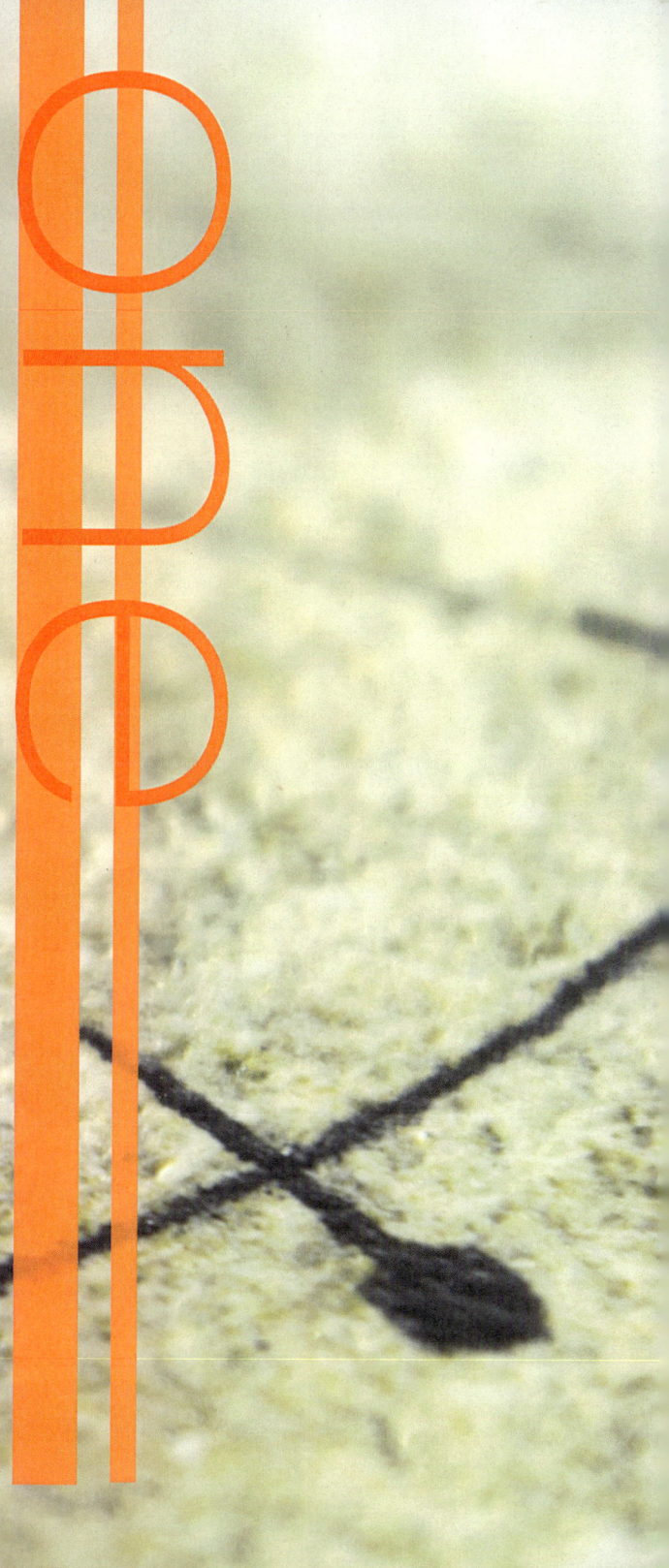

There are two moments in life that are more profound, more sacred than any other... Your very first breath and your last.

Without the first of these moments, you would never have lived the life you have lived. All the moments that followed and all the experiences you encountered would have never existed.

Without the second of these most profound moments your life would be without meaning, for it is through death that we find the value of life. Death means our life is finite. It is that final breath that makes all that we are, precious.

The challenge is we cannot remember our birth. That first breath was lost to both our inability to make memories at that time and to our incomprehension of the world. We did not have the mechanisms to define anything about that first breath, other than experiencing it as a brief and transitory feeling. A feeling we do not remember.

The other most profound of moments we will neverknow because it will arrive at a point in which we cease to exist. Death is not a part of life—it is a state that comes when life has ended.

As we head towards death, we enter the *Death Adventure*—a journey towards something other than life. In this journey, we can never truly know our destination because even if we glimpse that experience, we do so as a *living* thing. Only when life is no more can we fully know death. And at that point in time the death adventure is complete.

As such a mysterious and unknowable thing, death is to us like a grain of sand to an oyster. The oyster will wrap this irritation in layer upon layer of mucus, until it creates a beautiful pearl. This pearl is the investment of a lifetime's work and effort.

Our own death is the grain of sand; the irritant in which we invest our whole lifetime. Around that single point in time, we wrap layer upon layer of experiences. Moments that reflect and refract the light into a beautiful pearl—our legacy. This is a testament to the life we have lived and the moments we have made.

Without our last breath, none of this would happen. We would have no grain of sand around which to make the pearl of our lifetime. We would have no reason to cherish the finite time we have.

These two cornerstones of our existence do not just happen at the beginning and end of life—they define every moment of it! Who you were born to be and how you lived your entire life are at the core of everything you do: your motivations, personality, and achievements.

This lifetime (and every one of its moments) is so profound and limited that human culture has invested millennia attempting to understand it within the context of the universe and everything that exists beyond life. Culturally, spiritually and intellectually we seek to find reason, meaning and value in the blink of an eye we have.

Here and there, we catch a glimpse of the benevolence woven throughout our lifetime; of the one who values that pearl we create. The one who wears the necklace our pearl is an essential part of. The divine and eternal one who permeates every moment of our lifetime and of every other being.

So small our lives, so vast that benevolent force; we often get lost in the translation from one to the other. We fail to see the immensity of the divine within ourselves and so we lose the ability to act from a place of divinity within the minute passing of time. Instead, we settle on focusing on that which is small and petty in relation to the infinite, rather than cherishing the modest and invaluable, made precious by the infinite.

How we act in a moment defines how we live our lives. When you align your moments in pursuit of a greater purpose, you are honouring your first breath and also your last. Each experience comes to reflect and refract the core polarity of our lifetime. If you spend your time not valuing the core principles of your life, you create repetitive behaviours that make you uneasy.

A moment of legacy feels good, whilst a moment wasted causes frustration, anger, fear and a whole slew of other emotions that challenge and dishearten. Ultimately, we come to realise on some level that we are wasting life. We are not honouring our purpose. Our goal falls further beyond our grasp.

The growing sense of uneasiness eventually develops into dis-ease. Over time and repetition, the patterns of dis-ease cause habitual

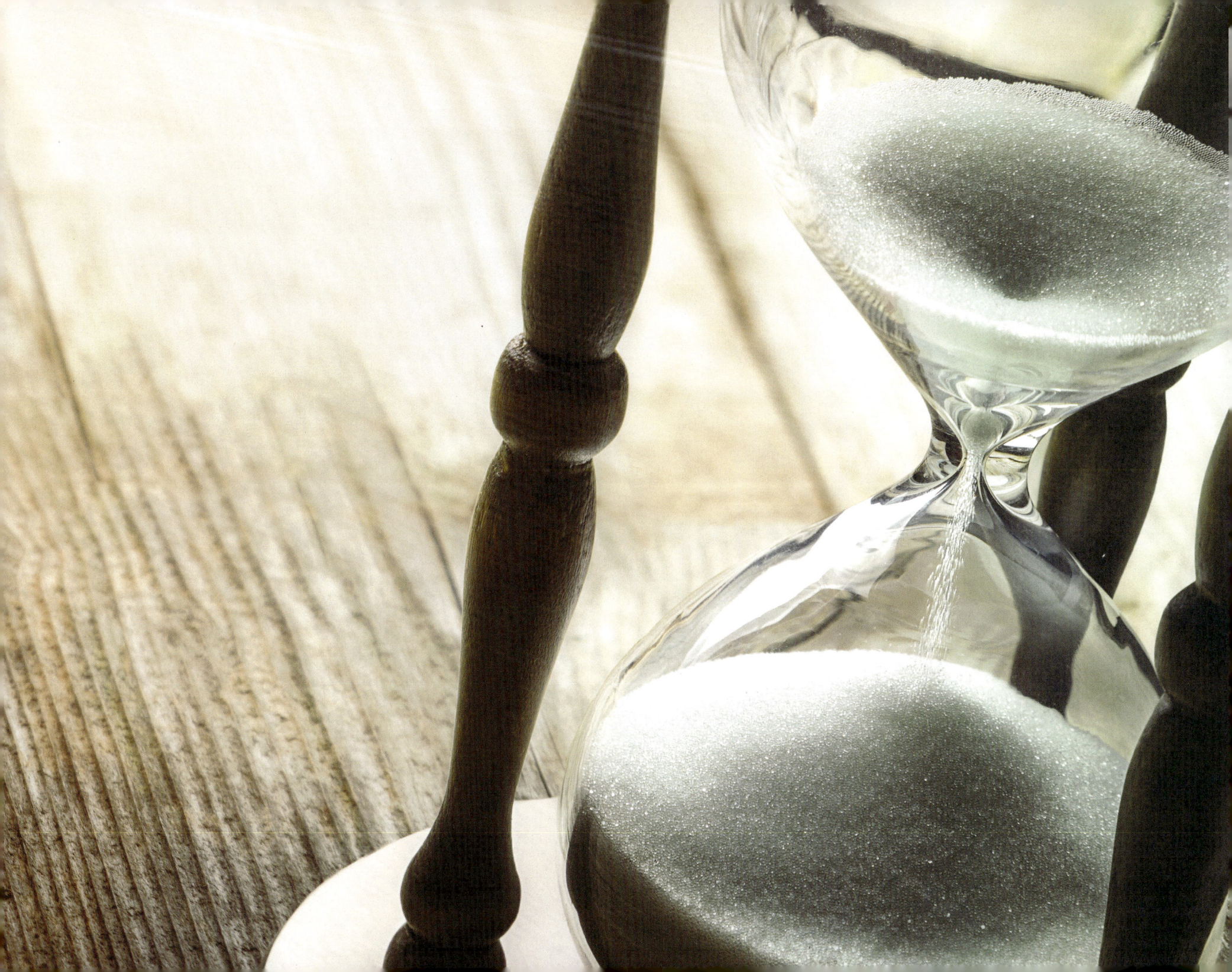

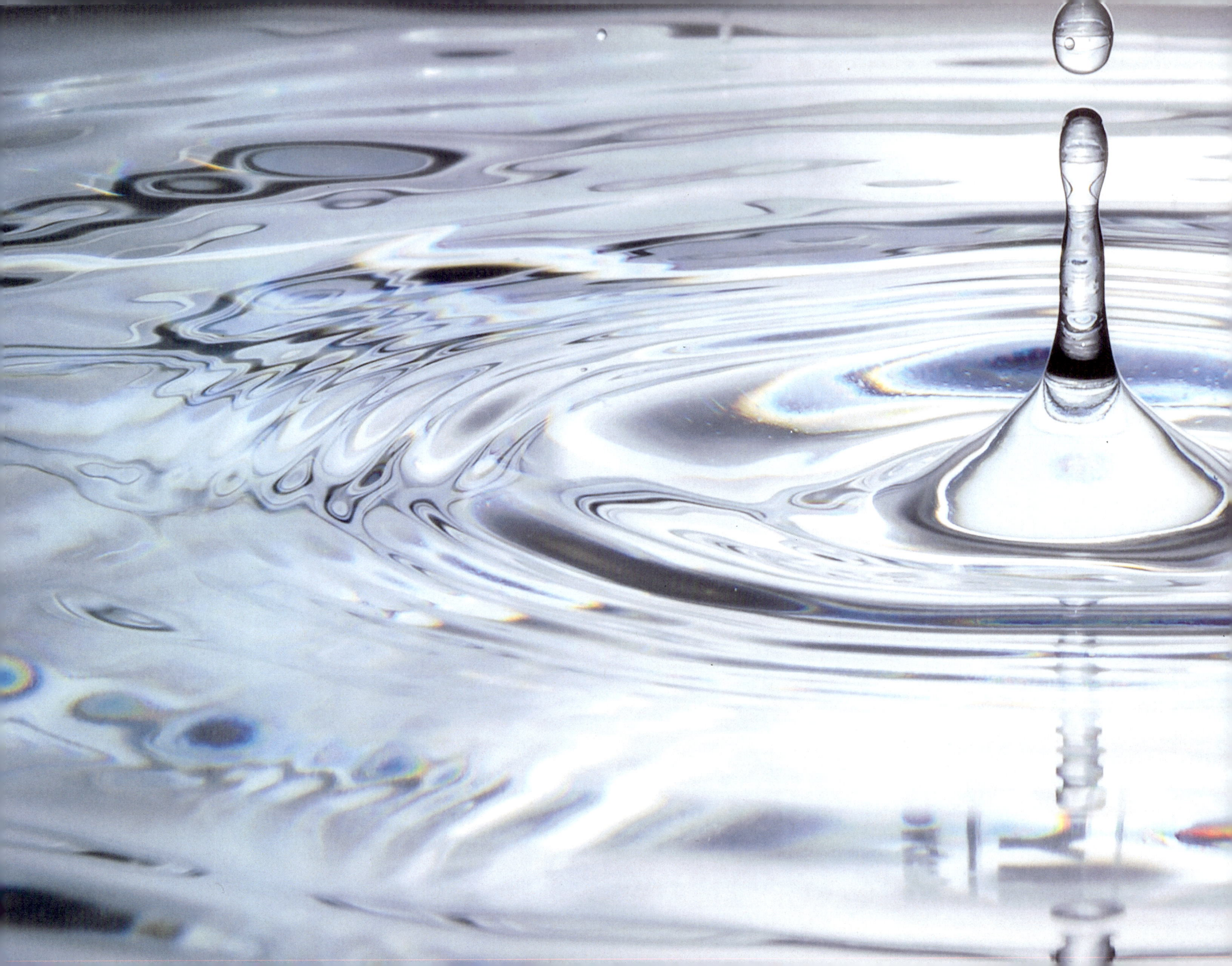

behaviours and we end up finding ourselves stuck in a perpetual pattern of behaviour and emotion; of reaction and reduction.

As the dis-ease gets worse we express this through different symptoms; some spiritual, some psychological, some emotional and some physical. Our lifetime, our birth, our death, and the pearl they create, become intrinsically tainted with dis-ease and that string of pearls becomes a testament of lifetimes of dis-ease, pain, and hardship, rather than the beauty it was intended to express.

This concept of many lives, expressed through time with dis-ease has spawned many contrasting philosophies, depending on the era, the culture, and the context. Unravelling the mysteries of these lives in relation to our own is a profound journey that offers lessons to be learnt and pain to be healed. One that we can take within the context of our own beliefs and perspective.

This philosophy is at the heart of *Karmic Regression Therapy*; seeking to use a framework that sits best with the individual being treated and leveraging that framework to heal through time. Essentially, KRT and its predecessor—*Karmic Reiki*—are therapies based on time, or the lack of it!

And this is reflected both in the origination of the therapy and in the act of treatment. As we wander through a cascading wealth of experiences—moments in time—and connect them to the current experience of our client, we are bending the core ethos of birth and death around this moment now.

Do these moments represent the lives we live? Are these moments from our ancestors' lives? Moments that many have encountered beyond the concept of the self? Or do these moments exist outside of time? The purpose of the multi-perspective view of KRT is to take the initial concept of *karma* and transition through several distinct viewpoints.

As you progress towards being a Karmic Regression therapist, you will no doubt find certain aspects of our journey make more sense to you than others. You will resonate with particular ideals and philosophies. However, the journey is *one journey* but seen through different perspectives. This offers us a wonderful starting point: we can speculate that the universe, in all its entirety and majesty, is merely one journey seen from many perspectives.

Karmic Reiki and Karmic Regression Therapy:

Therapies Developed Through Time

two

Karmic Reiki was the second therapy I originated from nothing. Whereas my first form of therapy, Celtic Reiki, was birthed from a single moment and specific experience, my sophomore effort developed through time and the experience of many moments.

This is not to say that Celtic Reiki was complete in a single moment. Two decades of continual refinement have led me to believe that Celtic Reiki will never be complete. Its development and refinement is an ongoing process. However, Celtic Reiki was planted with a single seed. Karmic Reiki was different. It came to me subtly through hundreds of treatment experiences and whilst working with many different clients.

Therefore, it is fitting to say that Celtic Reiki was made from an interaction and has come to represent the interactions of communities. Karmic Reiki and KRT have come to symbolise time and our perception of time.

With the development of One Therapy—my latest pioneering effort in the therapeutic profession—we envision how our universe and therapeutic journey in relation to the universe can be achieved through interaction, perception, dimension, space and time. In this context, KRT represents time.

Time is the greatest of all healers—it mends all wounds. Everything seems better with time.

However, time is also the creator of all wounds and pains. We experience hurt through time, without knowing how to heal it, until time unveils the solution to overcoming the pain. The solution to pain could be proactive—something you do—or simply the fading of pain over time, healing that just happens.

Imagine a world without time; a place where everything that ever was or will be exists concurrently. In the very same moment, you would experience both the pain and the healing of the pain. The two sides of the same experience would essentially negate each other.

Here, whilst feeling the pain, you would also feel the absence of pain. This would not only take away the pain but also the joy of overcoming the pain and the precious moments that we find in the journey between pain and healing. In a world without time we would feel no pain and no joy, just a sense of being numb.

During my years as a therapist and teacher I have worked with many different people, including people addicted to methamphetamine. Even though they were in a place of recovery, many of them would turn their back on sobriety from time to time. At first, it was unfathomable why a person would go anywhere near that particular drug, let alone relapse after witnessing first-hand the damage it causes.

Over time and through really listening to the people I met in Canadian drug support centres, I pieced together the common themes in their stories—how and why they are addicts and what causes them to turn their backs on sobriety so frequently.

When someone is marginalised by their community and society; when they are constantly told they are a freak, they are ugly, *going to burn in hell* because of who they were born to be, and so on, they are made to feel outsiders within their community and society. They internalise this hatred and seek to find a release from the constant, driving pain that stems from being ostracised.

Some turn to a network of supportive friends or find a new community or family. Others give meaning to their pain through fighting the good fight and turning their experiences into a powerful legacy for change. But some look to sex, food, alcohol and numbing the pain through brief and fleeting moments of pleasure.

Meth acts on the pleasure and reward part of the brain, in particular, the naturally occurring neurochemical, dopamine. Taking the drug rewards the user with a dose of dopamine that is hundreds of times greater than most people experience in a day. This is not only pleasurable; it provides something that is truly at the heart of why people become meth addicts...

The experience of all that dopamine offers the person a sense of self-acceptance that most people take for granted. Imagine you *know*, just for a moment, that you are not a freak; that you are attractive and are not going to burn in hell. Imagine feeling acceptable—equal to everybody else. Oftentimes, this sense of being human—just like everybody else—is at the heart of why people become addicts.

The clichéd view of a pleasure-seeking hedonist, shallow and just out for their next high, pales in comparison to the realisation that when someone first tries meth they are really looking for the mythical state of reality known as *normality*!

The challenge of meth is that it also destroys the production centres for dopamine. Therefore, people lose the ability to feel joy and reward very quickly. The only way they can get a sense of achievement or acceptance is to keep taking the drug. When they become sober, no effort of their own can bring back the sense of achievement or worth.

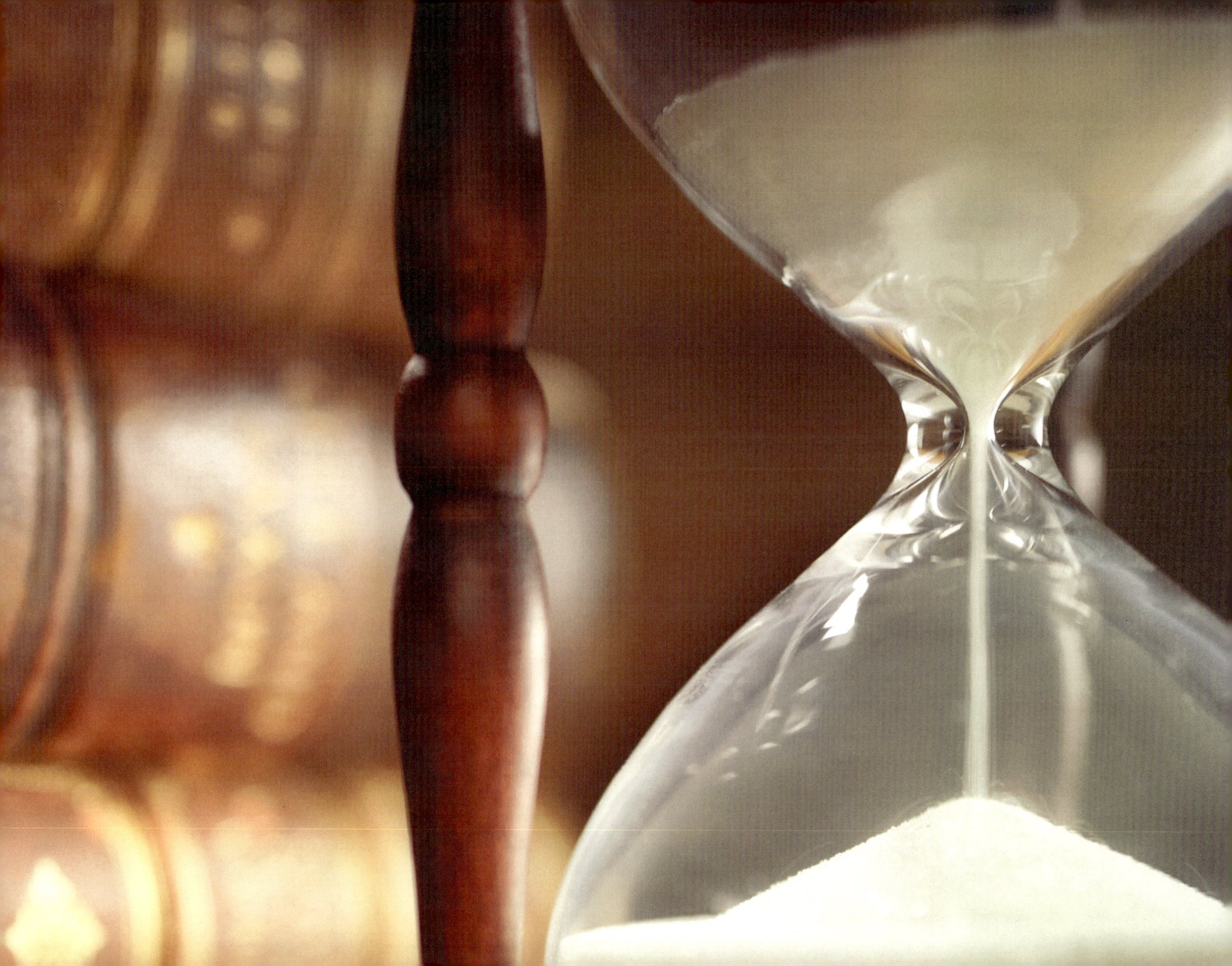

The pain becomes their normality and any sense of joy that could be there, is no more. This leads to a monotone existence; a sense of numbness, where being sober is just what others tell you is good.

There is no internal compass that lets them know they are doing a good job and reclaiming their health, life, and happiness. The only thing that does that is the drug.

Similarly; in a world without time, we would all feel that sense of numbness and ultimately lack any internal compass or sense of emotion. As pain and overcoming pain blur into a sensory mush, the only antidote to this state would be living through the experience of time.

Time provides a pause between pain and release; it enables us to attain a feeling of reward by counteracting the thing that caused us hurt in the first place. Time heals pain and also causes it—in order to heal it.

This simple ethos is the basis for an addiction almost everybody has: the addiction to time. We not only accept that time is the only reality there is, but seek to find more time, get more from it, and we see it as if it were *all we have.*

In the face of their death, people crave time. Many others, especially the young, squander time as if it were an endless resource. We devalue our time by giving it away to those who do not respect it. We also have a tendency to *spend* time, rather than *invest* it.

So, what happens when we break our addictive habits around time? Well, just as recovery from a meth addiction offers no pleasure, the time-detox leaves us in pain or just numb. However, unlike a meth addiction, we *can* change this. Becoming time-sober frees you to choose both the pain and the recovery from pain.

When we step outside of time, we realise that we have experienced pain many times over, in different situations, contexts, and circumstances. Yet, we have healed so little of it. This lack of healing encourages numbness or lack of feeling.

Over time, we have just let the pain fade into a sense of normality—as if the pain is how things should be, instead of an obstacle to be removed. The moment you turn a time-detox into a proactive healing strategy that exists beyond time, you begin to reap the rewards; the solutions to age-old trauma that is just stuck there, through time, without resolution.

Should a person in time encounter a traumatic event that affects them profoundly, their whole world shifts to a different level of experience. Although people who go to war, suffer a crippling disease or terrible loss *can* move forward, they are usually haunted by what they experienced.

Without the healing from the trauma, and whilst they are still in a world formed by the trauma, they find similar or worse iterations of those experiences. Living trapped in the world of suffering—without actively transitioning into the place where the trauma is healed—causes a lifetime of repeating cycles.

When we turn our attention to both karma and miasma, we realise that these cycles extend beyond death. Through the karmic journey of the soul, karmic patterns, and our own ancestry, we may be *born* into a world of trauma—one that was created in another lifetime.

Many people live their entire lives in a repeating cycle—fighting battles, suffering from terrible illness, and bearing the weight of excruciating pain; be it emotional, physical or psychological.

Without knowing the specific cause, they may never solve the puzzle of where the trauma was originated. Or, they may blame the first experience of an ever-repeating cycle. Here, a person will focus on an event, usually from childhood, and assume that it is the cause of their problems, when that particular event is just a continuation of much older dynamics.

The good news is, the trauma has already been created; all that is required to break the cycle is to actively heal oneself and to learn how that journey unfolds—transcending the karmic event, breaking the karmic pattern or re-patterning the miasmatic effects of the trauma.

The most common situation I have encountered in consultation sessions is that people continue to work through similar themes of trauma or dis-ease, which they believe have been healed but keep coming back in some other way (as if they are experiencing the same root issue, but from a different perspective).

Looking back over the years, Karmic Reiki and Karmic Regression Therapy have grown not from any one incident, but are a gradual synthesis of treatments, consultations, and feedback, combined with the situations I have encountered and the people I have met along the way.

This journey—my journey—exists through time and beyond time. It is both the tale of a therapy created and a life lived. I can access these memories as conscious experiences, but I can also access the vibrations and driving force behind this journey: the miasma and karma of the moments invested within KRT.

Thus, our therapy of time is mirrored within time, through time, and in an eternal state outside of time. As each moment that

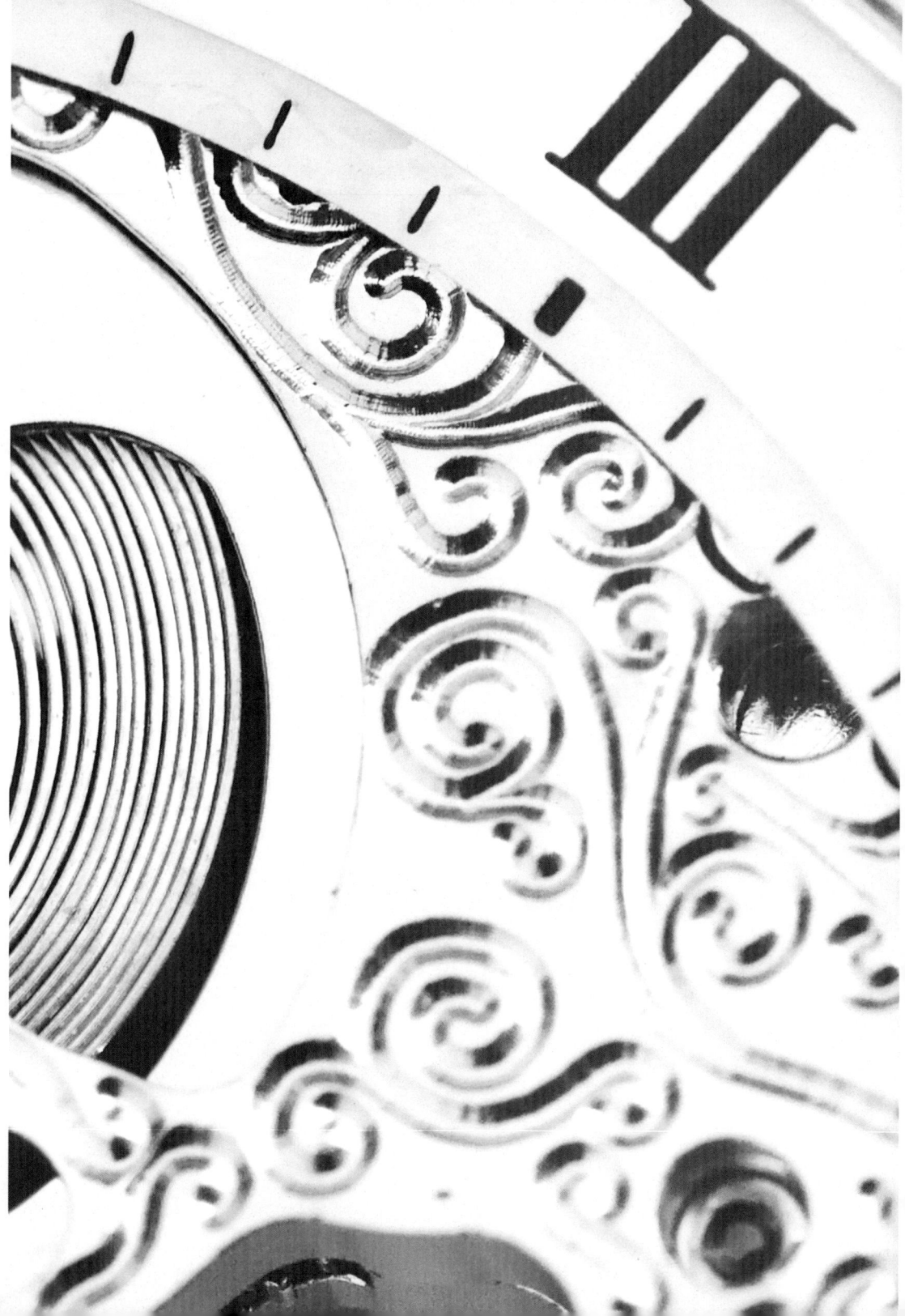

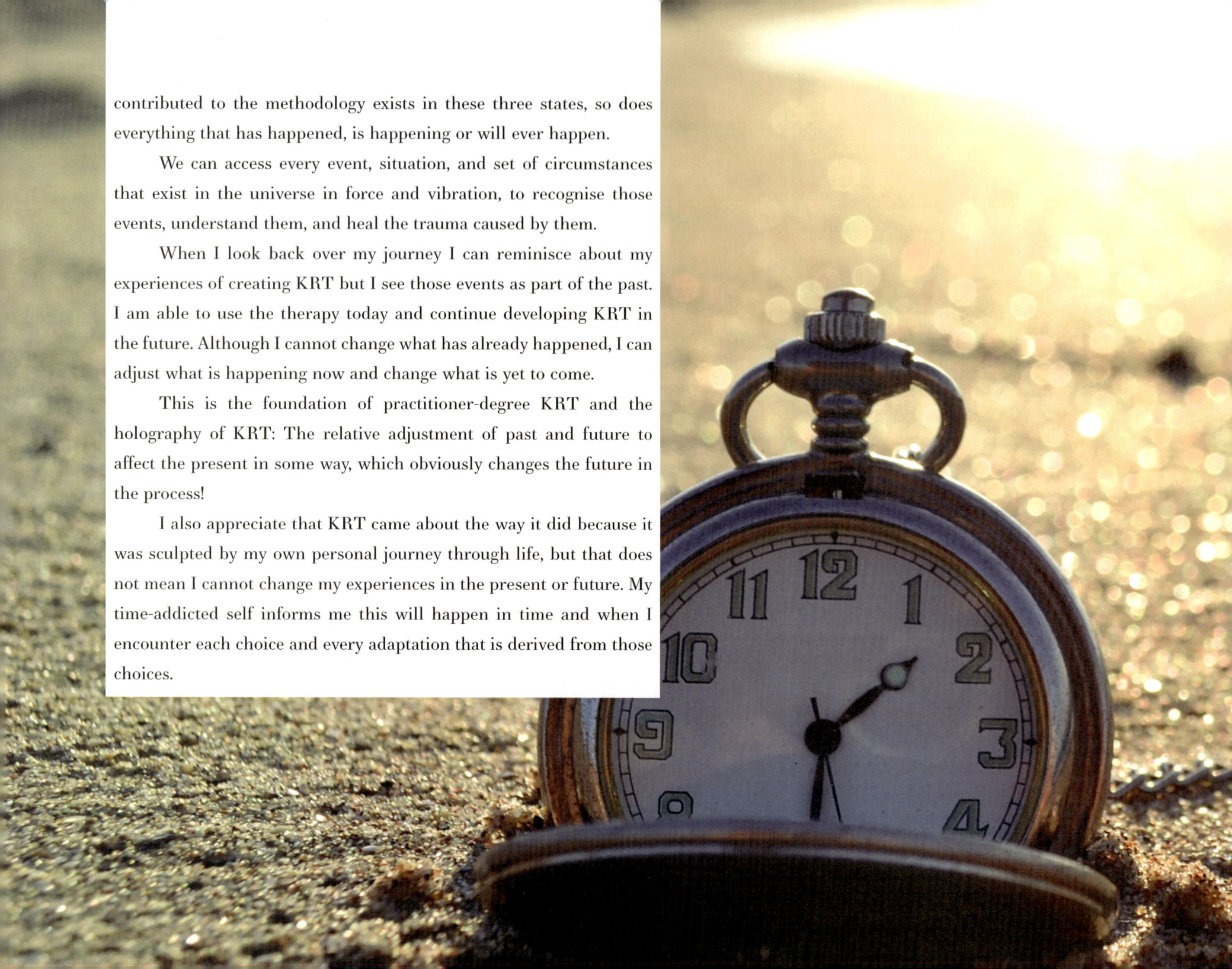

contributed to the methodology exists in these three states, so does everything that has happened, is happening or will ever happen.

We can access every event, situation, and set of circumstances that exist in the universe in force and vibration, to recognise those events, understand them, and heal the trauma caused by them.

When I look back over my journey I can reminisce about my experiences of creating KRT but I see those events as part of the past. I am able to use the therapy today and continue developing KRT in the future. Although I cannot change what has already happened, I can adjust what is happening now and change what is yet to come.

This is the foundation of practitioner-degree KRT and the holography of KRT: The relative adjustment of past and future to affect the present in some way, which obviously changes the future in the process!

I also appreciate that KRT came about the way it did because it was sculpted by my own personal journey through life, but that does not mean I cannot change my experiences in the present or future. My time-addicted self informs me this will happen in time and when I encounter each choice and every adaptation that is derived from those choices.

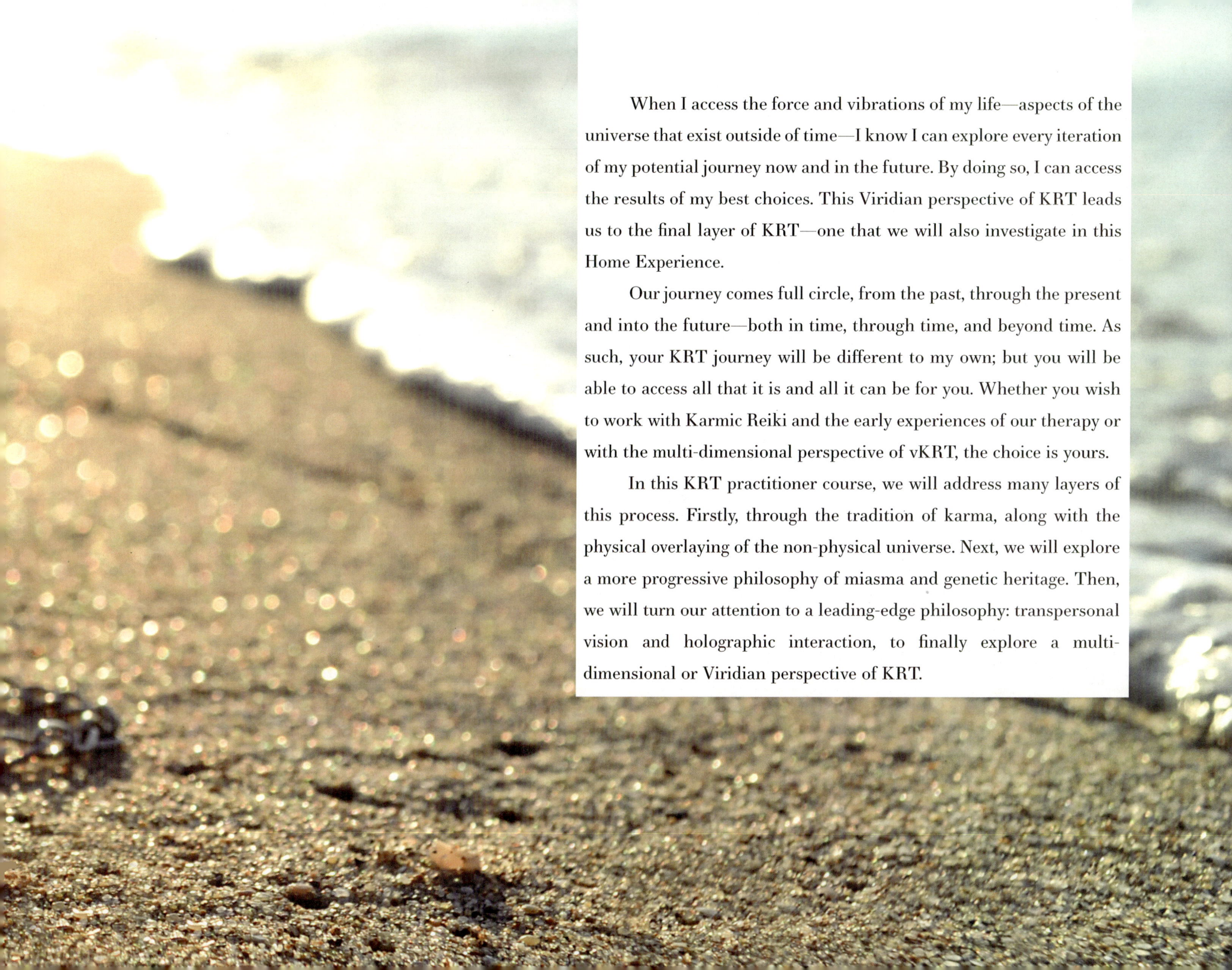

When I access the force and vibrations of my life—aspects of the universe that exist outside of time—I know I can explore every iteration of my potential journey now and in the future. By doing so, I can access the results of my best choices. This Viridian perspective of KRT leads us to the final layer of KRT—one that we will also investigate in this Home Experience.

Our journey comes full circle, from the past, through the present and into the future—both in time, through time, and beyond time. As such, your KRT journey will be different to my own; but you will be able to access all that it is and all it can be for you. Whether you wish to work with Karmic Reiki and the early experiences of our therapy or with the multi-dimensional perspective of vKRT, the choice is yours.

In this KRT practitioner course, we will address many layers of this process. Firstly, through the tradition of karma, along with the physical overlaying of the non-physical universe. Next, we will explore a more progressive philosophy of miasma and genetic heritage. Then, we will turn our attention to a leading-edge philosophy: transpersonal vision and holographic interaction, to finally explore a multi-dimensional or Viridian perspective of KRT.

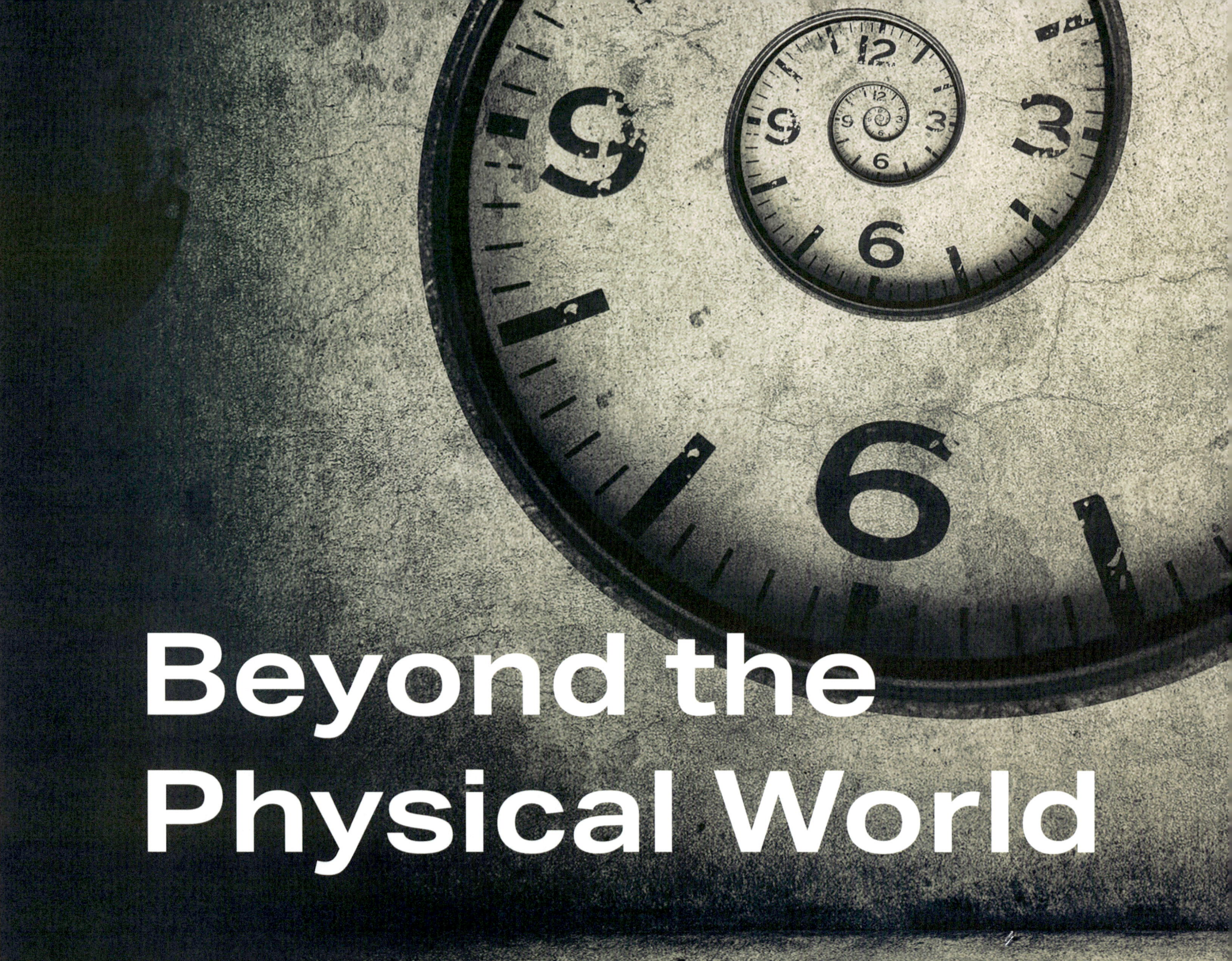

Beyond the Physical World

For thousands of years, humankind has speculated about what exists beyond the physical world.

For millennia, this spiritual adventure has defined cultures and societies, inspiring a broad array of art, philosophy, law and even science.

Yet, the principles behind much of our definition of the spiritual realm are based on taking our sensory perceptions of the world and *overlaying* them on to the non-physical universe. A god that looks like a man, energy that travels from one place to another, etheric beings that are motivated by human emotion, gender-based archetypes, and so on.

I hold a rather controversial view: that the physical world is but a sliver of an incomprehensible and infinite universe: a universe that, by definition, cannot be compared to the physical world, although it is experienced through the physical. This non-physical universe transcends the concepts of the three-dimensional (length, width, height), in addition to space and time.

The initial challenge we face is that our language is based upon these physical concepts, so communicating the non-physical reality is immediately challenging. Energy does not go from here to there; God is neither male, nor female, and they (not she or he) did not create the Earth at some distant point in the past, because the past is an illusion of the physical world.

Spirit is not up or down, nothing travels in a circle, and everything is a part of one giant whole, without separation or distinction other than a few physical world definitions. You and I, therefore, are a quirk of physicality, and these words you are reading exist as a definition of physicality in their own right. They simply exist as a thought, extending across the illusory idea of two people.

In recent history, a massive polarisation has developed in the physical world, between people who put their faith in the physical world and those who have faith beyond it. This polarity is a source of great conflict, to the point where an all-encompassing paradigm-shift is inevitable. The physical world is based on polarity—it is a necessary part of the universal fabric because without two forces acting upon each other, there is nothing to contrast one thing from another.

This shift will help us gain a deeper understanding of the processes of the non-physical universe—where we define ourselves with a greater degree of complexity and dynamism. However, as we transform within, the perception of the past, present, and future still creates conflict within us. Here we discover the foundations of Karmic Regression Therapy.

From a non-physical perspective, everything exists in balance and harmony—it simply is.

In physicality, our memory of the past, perception of the present, and choices that spur future actions provide linear continuity to our lives. We remember, we experience and we project into the illusion of our future.

If we were to look at the universe as if it were a book, then every chapter and every word exists perfectly as it should, from opening paragraph to last word. Here, the reader of that book is the physical-world journey we take through the experience of that book, just as every living thing goes on an adventure through the universe.

When reading a book, each reader remembers what has happened, perceives the words as they pass in front of them and wonders what will come next. However, the book exists—in its entirety—regardless of what we remember, what we perceive, or what we hope will happen.

Before we actually read the book, it exists. Afterwards, it exists. Whilst we are reading it, the book exists as something complete. There is a difference between the *constant* state of the book and our conscious interaction with it. Whilst the book exists on its own, our conscious experience *transitions* from the possibility of reading it, to the journey of reading it and the memory of having read it, and then back to the possibility of re-reading it, with the added knowledge of our previous experience.

The experiences and lessons we learn by reading the book, are rather like the events, situations and circumstances we encounter through life. These experiences exist regardless of our

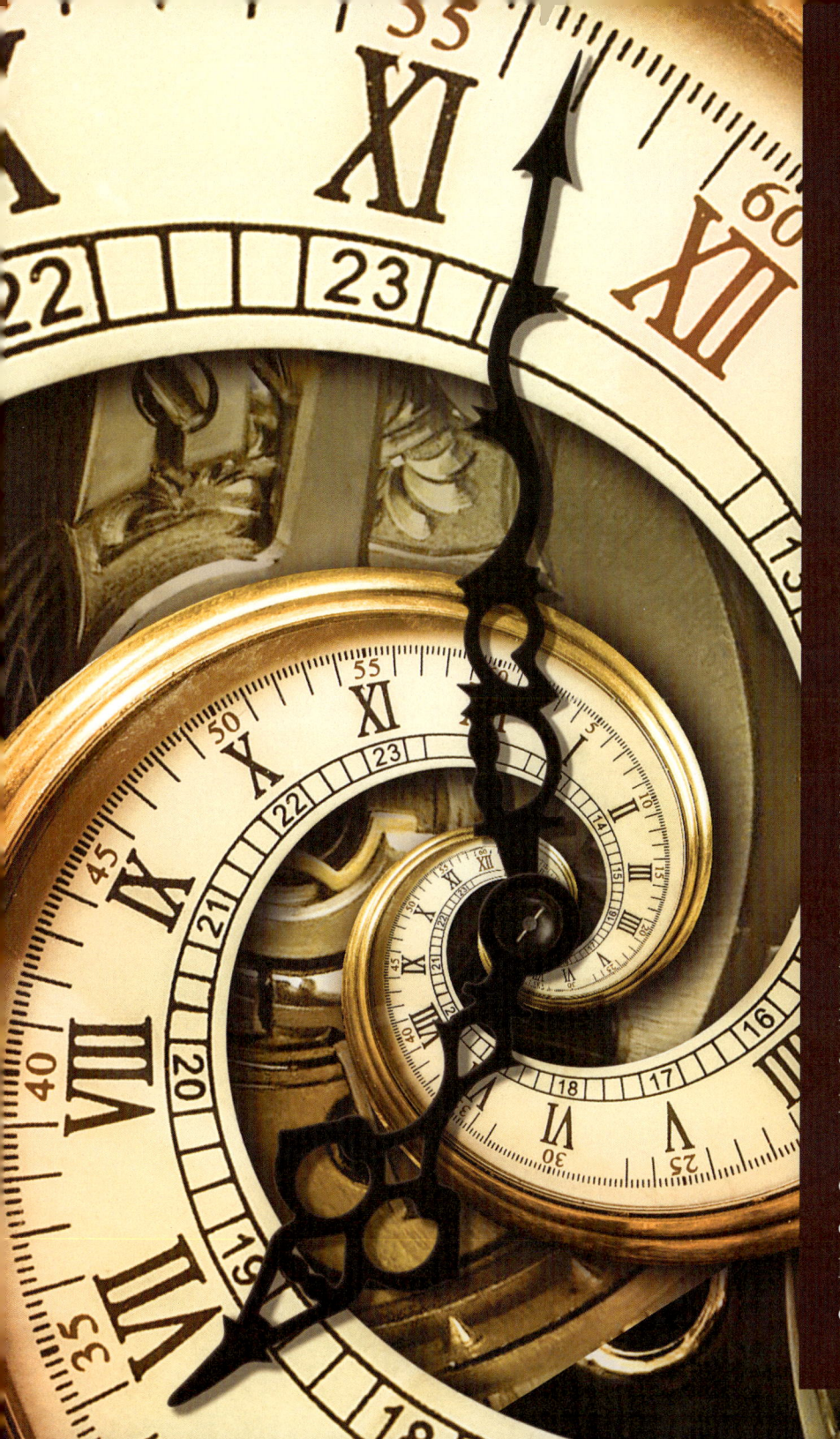

choices and actions. However, it is not until we become consciously aware of their existence that they become part of our lifetime.

Once we become aware of a particular narrative in the universe, the impact it has is so powerful at a personal level that we tend to go back and re-experience that narrative time and time again. This goes on to the point that we cannot even remember the initial event that started the chain. The original event becomes lost in time; fading in some other lifetime, but the pattern of behaviour it started, remains.

This is what we know as a *karmic pattern*. There are many different karmic patterns, which include: anger, jealousy, apathy, narcissism, hedonism and so on. We might fall into a sensation of being invisible and having no effect in the world. We may become a victim to bullies or power abusers. In most circumstances, any of the karmic patterns we are compelled to recreate and perpetuate are but single threads in a complex tapestry of time and consciousness.

Keep in mind that when we create a karmic pattern, it is a *transpersonal* experience, regardless of how personal it feels. If we do something out of anger, it does not mean it is your anger—it is just anger. Being driven by jealousy does not mean you are a jealous person. Instead, think of this as performing the karmic pattern of jealousy.

We may even go as far as to say that when you are consciously recreating a karmic pattern, you are in the service of that particular pattern. And anybody who demonstrates that karma is working from the same pattern as everybody who is connected to that karma.

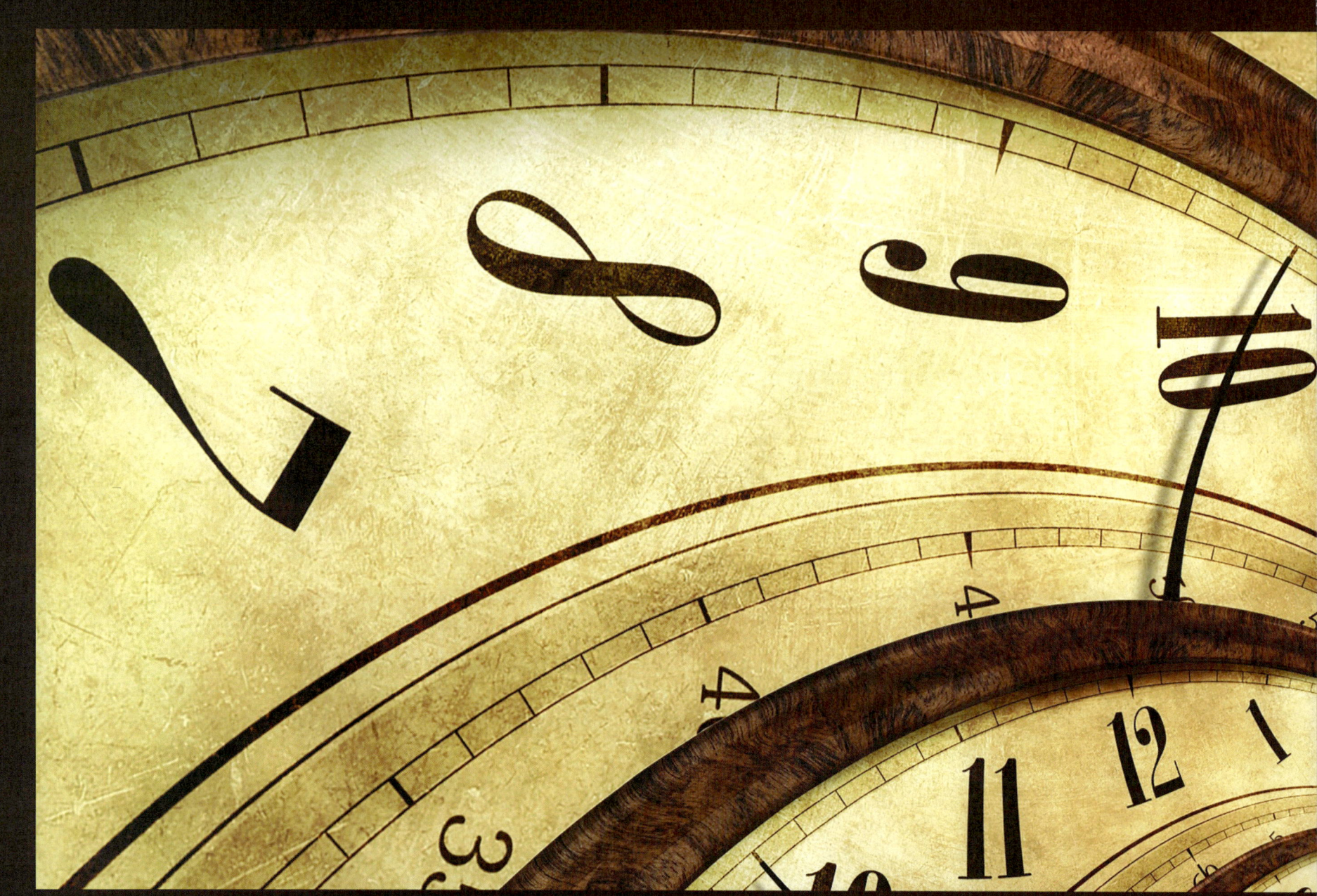

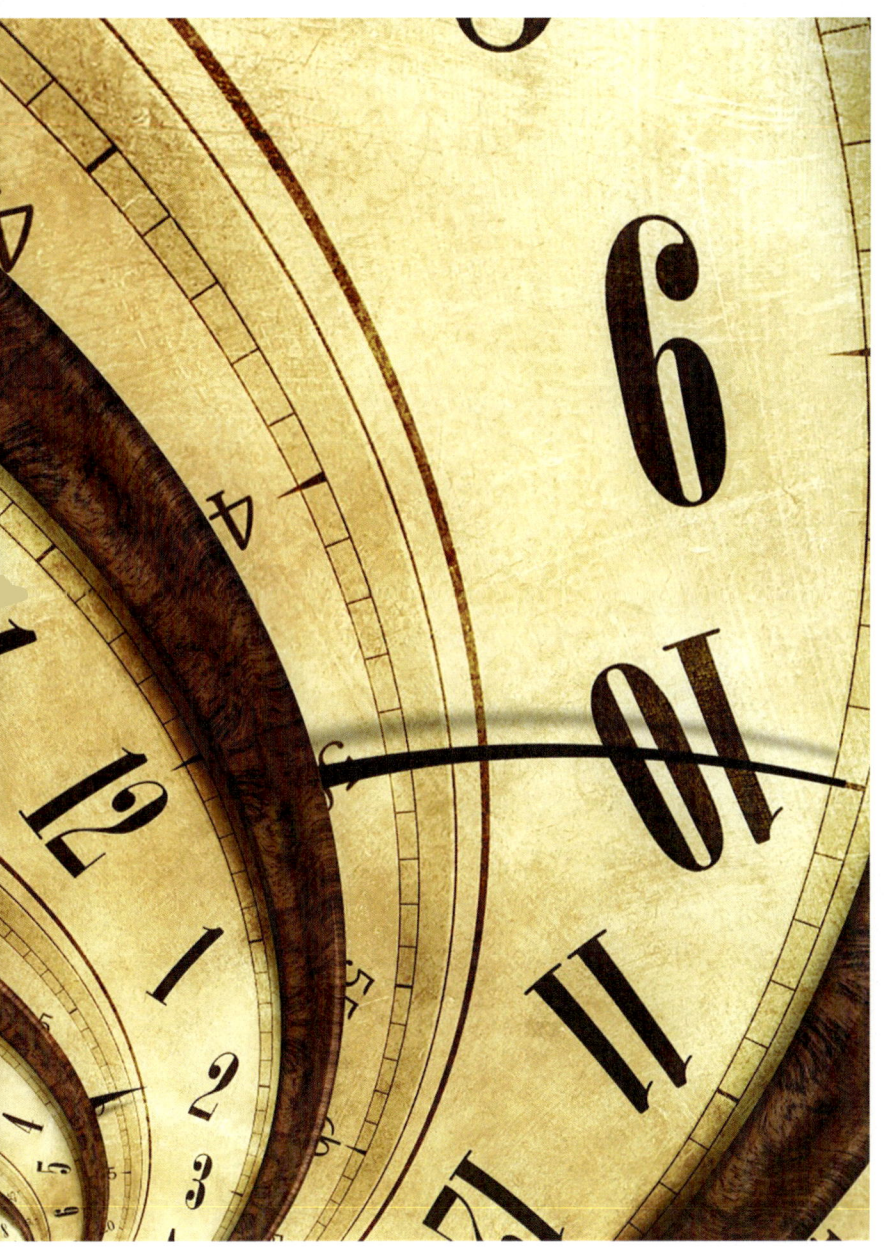

This is why we experience thresholds or gateways to karmic patterns. One minute you are experiencing a minor irritation at someone or something. Then, you reach a point where you know you can either let it go or you can push that feeling further. The moment you push further into that feeling, a minor annoyance is transformed into an overwhelming rage. It is as if the floodgates opened and all the hatred in the world spilled out.

The transpersonal or collective nature of karmic patterns means that we not only experience them personally but also as groups—ranging from small communities to society as a wider context. We can see this, for example, in groups of people with an endemic apathy towards achievement, or communities who spite themselves through pride.

Even entire generations of people are viewed as self-entitled, hedonistic, cruel or victimised. Karmic patterns affect us in our own, internal microcosm and in the wider, external macrocosm of the world.

Karmic patterns exist beyond our physical reality, yet on each occasion we connect into a pattern, it affects us emotionally, psychologically, spiritually and physically.

For some people, this is a question of reincarnation through many lives—a cycle of births, deaths, and rebirths. For others, it is more a question of ancestry—the miasma that stems from our heritage and continues as part of our ongoing legacy.

There are more complex and subtle perspectives of damaging patterns and how they are ingrained in our society—traditionally, politically, socially, in the media, and even in the way we communicate through language. Karma, in all its many forms and labels, saturates our lives. Our only way forward is committing to a time-detox, to identifying the karmic patterns we are working from, to healing holistically, and going forward, to making better choices.

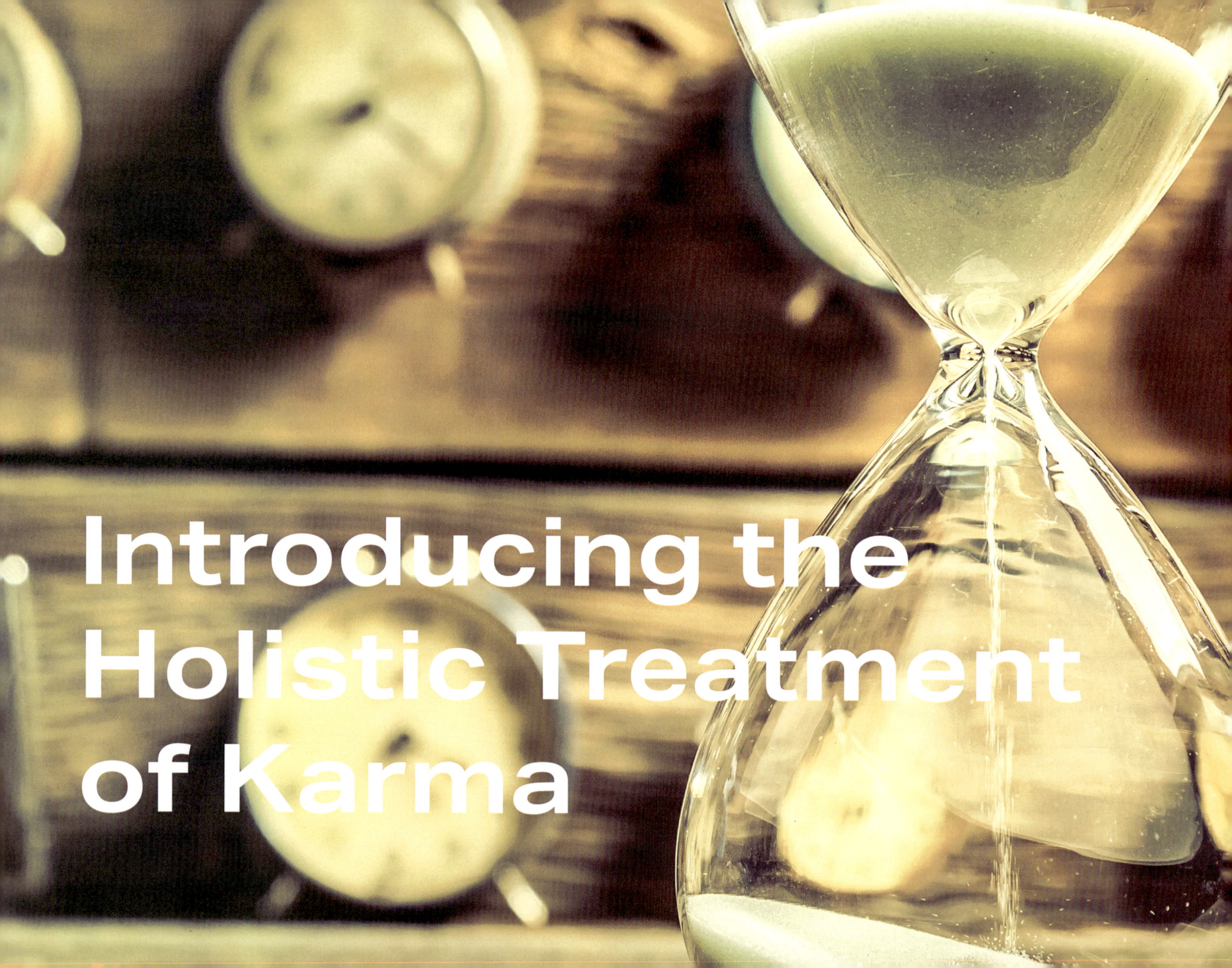

Introducing the Holistic Treatment of Karma

There are five distinct layers of Karmic Reiki/Karmic Regression Therapy methodology which form the practitioner degree of therapeutic practice. They are:

Karmic Reiki—The Soul's Journey through Time (Karmic Objects and Events)
Karmic Regression Therapy (Foundation Degree)—Karmic Patterns
mKRT—Miasmatic Regression/Vibrational Heritage
Holo-KRT—Holographic Patterns
vKRT (Practitioner Degree)—The Viridian or Non-Temporal Perspective of KRT

As you explore the Home Experience in further detail through this manual, the digital Realm Experience and the *Official Guide to KRT* book, you will discover the vast scope and power of KRT when it is applied professionally to help your clients.

In the initial week of exploration, you are guided to various resources in the realms and to specific chapters of the *Official Guide* book. These sources will help you take your first tentative steps into the Karmic experience.

Moving beyond the basic ethos of Karmic Reiki and KRT, you will need to explore the *Orientation and Calibration* process. Firstly, through self-calibration and then, through guided calibration. Once you have conducted at least one calibration session, you will be ready to begin testing the preparatory tools and techniques of Karmic Reiki.

Now, as Karmic Reiki developed out of Usui Reiki treatment sessions, we shall begin with some Usui Reiki practices, both traditional and modern.

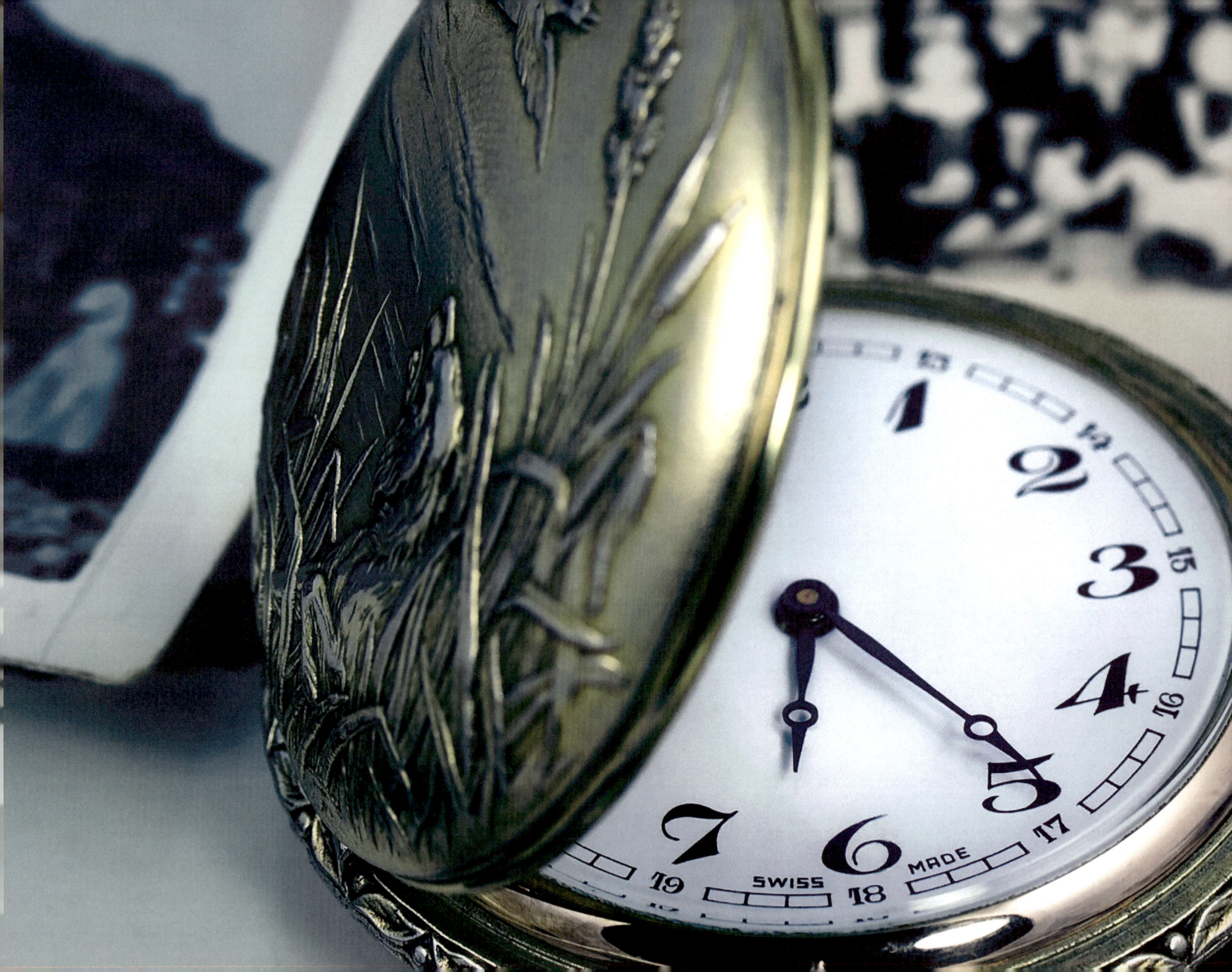

The first techniques we need to work with are two methods of treatment known as *Reiji Ho* and *Byosen Reikan Ho*. These ancient forms of practice were cornerstones of *Usui Teate*—the earliest known form of Reiki therapy modality, as originated by Mikao Usui.

Many practitioners in the West regard Usui as the father of Reiki therapeutic practices. His *Reiki Teate* forms the basis of many modern forms of Reiki therapy, including Karmic Reiki. For further information about Reiki and Reiki therapies, please see the mPowr *Reiki Revolution Home Experience* at *www.vreiki.com*.

These two therapeutic techniques—*Reiji Ho and Byosen Reikan Ho*—enable you to increase your sensitivity to the various sensations around your client's body. Being able to distinguish and interpret these sensations via your hands will, in turn, develop your intuitive ability.

Byosen Reikan Ho is used to monitor disruptions (known as *byosen*) in the area surrounding a person. Once detected, these disruptions can be removed, reduced or altered. This will enable healing throughout the body and beyond. By conducting regular and long-term Byosen Reikan Ho practice with many different people, it is possible for you to develop highly-refined sensitivity skills.

Byosen are said to be transmitted from the source or core of a person's dis-ease, illness or injury and can be felt in (or around) the hands of the practitioner. The sensation (known as *hibiki* or *resonance*) will depend on the variety, source and strength of the byosen, common descriptions of it include: "an insect crawling across the skin" or "a small coil springing across the practitioner's hand." Other hibiki include pain, numbness, heat, coldness, tickling, tingling, etc.

Byosen are said to appear a few days before symptoms develop and may still be detectable after the dis-ease has passed. This effect can indicate that the person may develop the symptoms again. For this reason, you may still experience byosen even if your client is in *perfect health*. This also implies that you can treat the a byosen to stop the disease from ever (re)appearing.

What you sense with each hibiki will depend on the cause and status of the disease, as well as the time it will take to heal. The presence of a byosen in a specific area does not necessarily mean that the dis-ease is located in the same physical area, as each byosen may appear in a completely different place from the actual infirmity.

What is important when sensing the byosen is to relax, clear your mind, and work with each byosen in detail, really honing your awareness on the sensations in your hand.

To conduct a treatment using Byosen Reikan Ho, you need to ensure that your client is laying comfortably on the treatment table. Start by sitting at the head-end of the table and connecting to your client. This is done through a *head connection*—place your hands either side of your client's head, palms facing inwards, as if you are holding an invisible ball around the client's head.

When you are ready, stand at either side of the table and use your non-dominant hand to *scan* the body of the client, sensing the hibiki of byosen in the air surrounding them (this can be from a few inches to several feet away).

Once you have discovered a byosen, treat the area until your awareness of the hibiki ceases or after ten minutes have passed. After clearing the byosen, repeat the scanning until you have located and cleared as many byosen as possible in time allotted to the treatment session.

Complete the treatment with a final head connection and, finally, bring your client's awareness back into the room.

Byosen Reikan Ho is a cerebral activity that requires the conscious scanning of your client. The approach of Reiji Ho is different, as it is conducted in a completely intuitive way. As the practitioner, you do not need to be aware of the dis-ease or issue and its relevant treatment because the entire process is performed intuitively.

To some people, Reiji Ho comes naturally. To others, it requires lots of practice. Oftentimes, people who instinctively take to Reiji Ho feel that mastering Byosen Reikan Ho is a challenging experience for them, and vice versa—although this is not always the case.

Regardless of the natural ability or affinity to either technique, both Reiji Ho and Byosen Reikan Ho are cornerstones of Reiki tradition and mastering them requires regular practice.

The Reiji Ho style of treatment uses a freeform movement of the hands to trace various dynamics around a client's body. To conduct a Reiji Ho treatment, start with a head connection and affirm mentally that you are going to treat your client with Reiji Ho. When you feel a good connection, move to the side

of the treatment table and place your hands over your client's abdominal region.

Practitioners of KRT who use Reiji Ho simply rest their hands on the invisible blanket of magnetic force that seems to extend away from the client's body. Just by holding this position in a very relaxed way, their hands will begin to move before long. Gradually, their hands begin to move to new positions.

For students who are new to this technique, this can be a little disconcerting. So, it is important not to make a change happen, or to resist the movement when it does—just go with the flow! If your hands move to their fullest extent, feel free to travel around your subject to reach a more comfortable position for yourself.

Remain at each position until your hands move again, of their own accord. Then, at the end of the treatment, go to your client's head area and finish with a head connection.

You can discover demonstrations of both Reiji Ho and Byosen Reikan Ho in the digital realms of the KRT Home Experience. Although these are only basic methods within Karmic Reiki, it is important to feel confident in both techniques before attempting any of the other, more elaborate treatment methods.

Whilst practising the styles of Reiji Ho and Byosen Reikan Ho and, therefore, increasing your sensory and intuitive skills, it is worth exploring the physiology behind these treatment methods. There are two different perspectives to consider here— the traditional Eastern philosophies of energy therapy anatomy and the modern, Western view of anatomy.

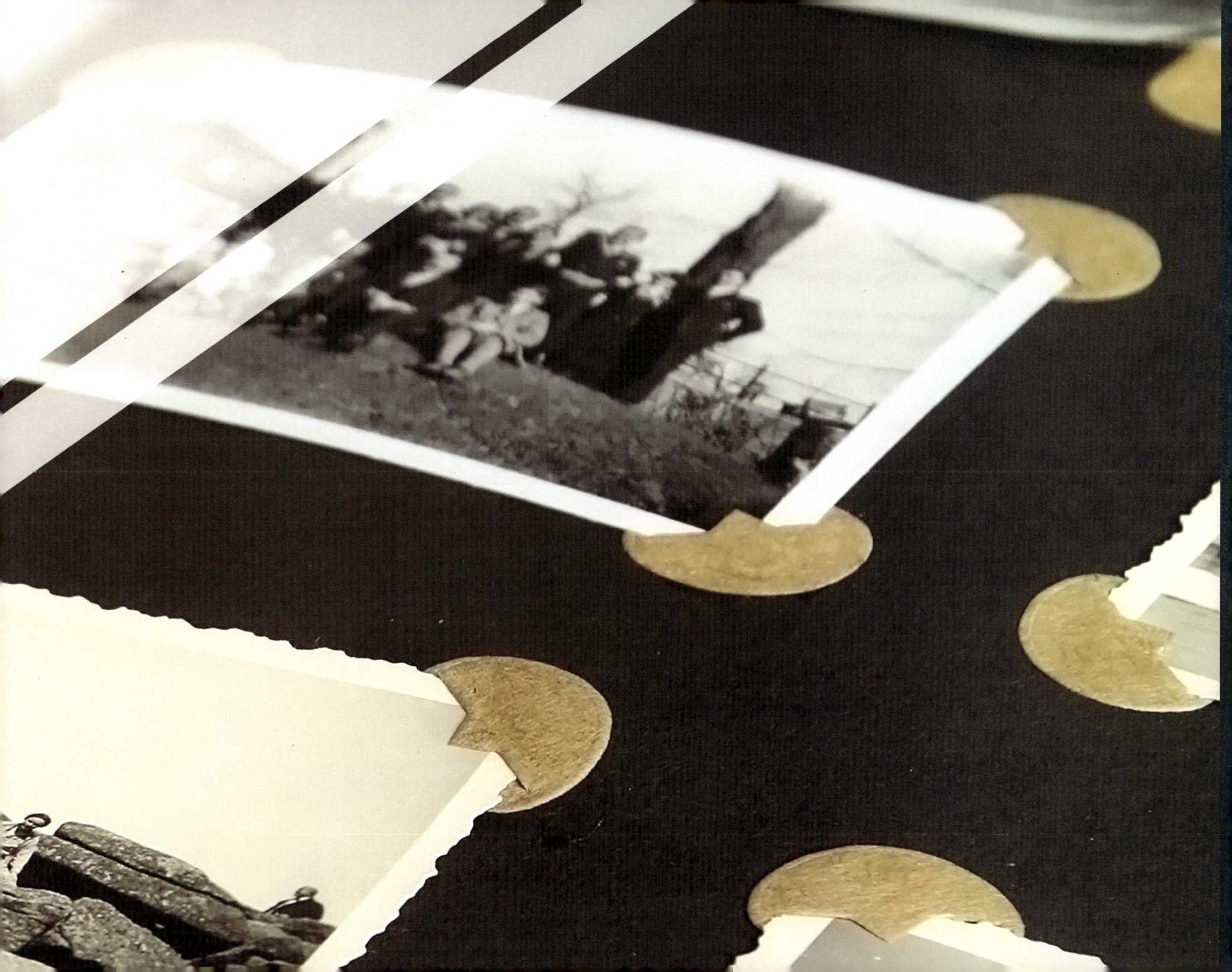

In the second week of training you will explore these physiological elements in much greater detail. But, for now, let us take a whirlwind tour of the Eastern view (*chakras, meridians* and the *aura*), with the addition of some more Western, scientific considerations (receptor bundles, the living matrix, and quantum philosophy).

The Sanskrit word *chakra* means *spinning wheel.* This illustrates very well the gyrating vortices of force that create the individual chakras! Traditionally, these whirlpools of energy are said to be a mysterious force known as *prana.*

The concept of prana comes from South Asia. Prana is seen as the force that creates and sustains all things, including life. Hence, each chakra is the point of prana transmission from the external world to the internal body and vice versa.

The type of prana being drawn in or released by a single chakra depends on each specific chakra. There are hundreds of chakras, most of which are known as *minor chakras.* However, in Reiki therapies we deal with nine main chakras and two pairs of minor chakras.

These are the Crown, Brow, Throat, Heart, Solar Plexus, Sacral, Base, Soul Star, Earth Star, The Palm chakras and the Foot chakras.

The vortex of each chakra is believed to spin in a particular direction and is located at on a specific point on the body. The main chakras are positioned at the base of the spine, below the navel, just below the ribcage, on the middle (or heart) area of the chest, on the base of the throat, on the brow and on the top of the head.

Each of these chakras is also associated with a particular colour, ranging from red at the base to white or violet at the crown. We need to absolutely stress one thing about working with the chakras: there is no definitive answer as to the location, colour or even the existence of chakras.

This is important to keep in mind because there is so much conflicting information and so many people with rigid opinions about the chakras that it is easy to become confused.

Some will say the chakras spin this way, others will say they all spin different ways. Some say the throat chakra is blue, while others affirm it's orange. Some people will show you a photo of their own chakras, even when no camera can actually take a picture of chakras because they are etheric and not physical!

Based on years of my own research, my perspective is that chakras are subjective. They exist in locations, rotations and a spectrum that are unique to each practitioner. Therefore, whilst your perspective is essential for you, others may have a different experience—and that's okay!

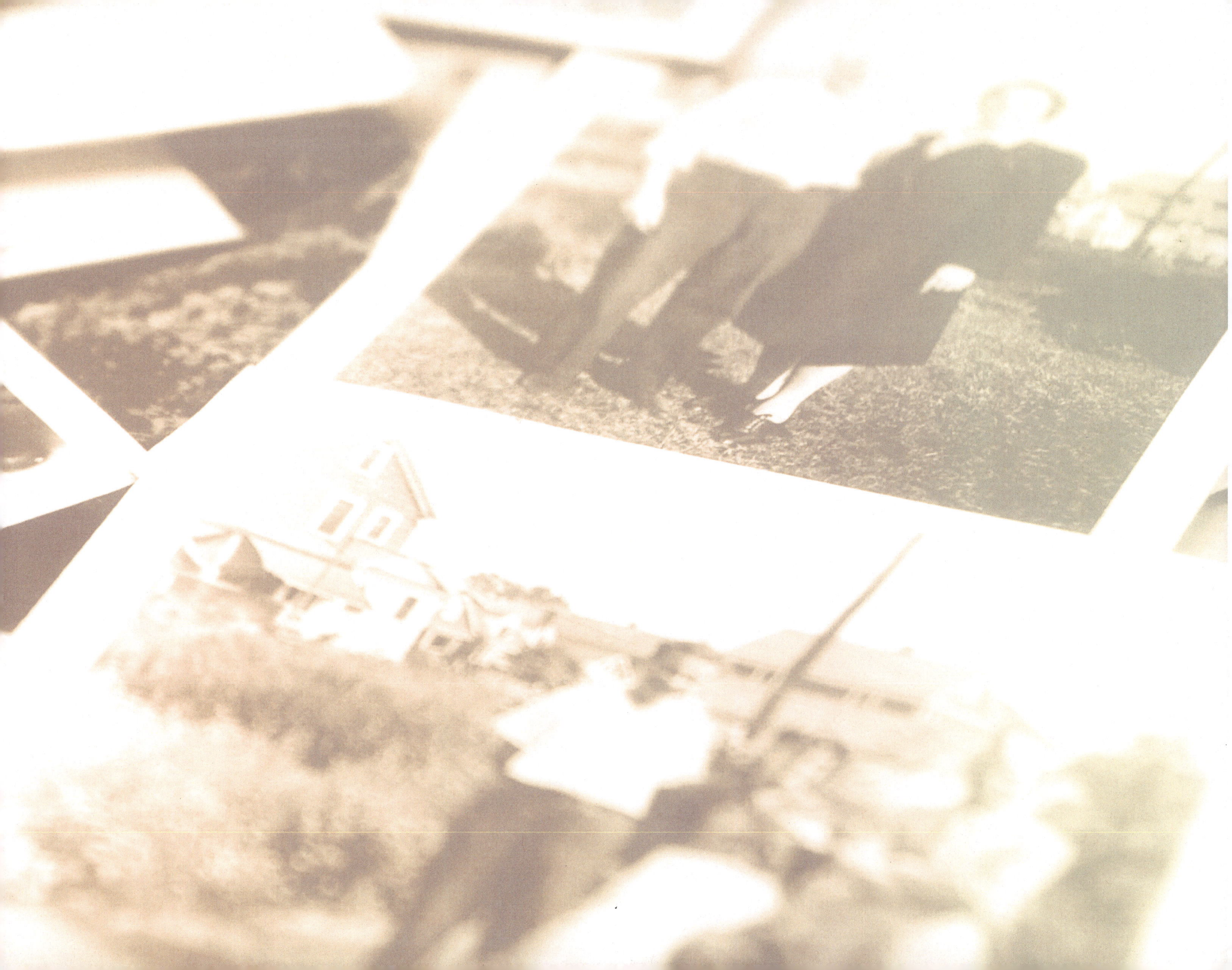

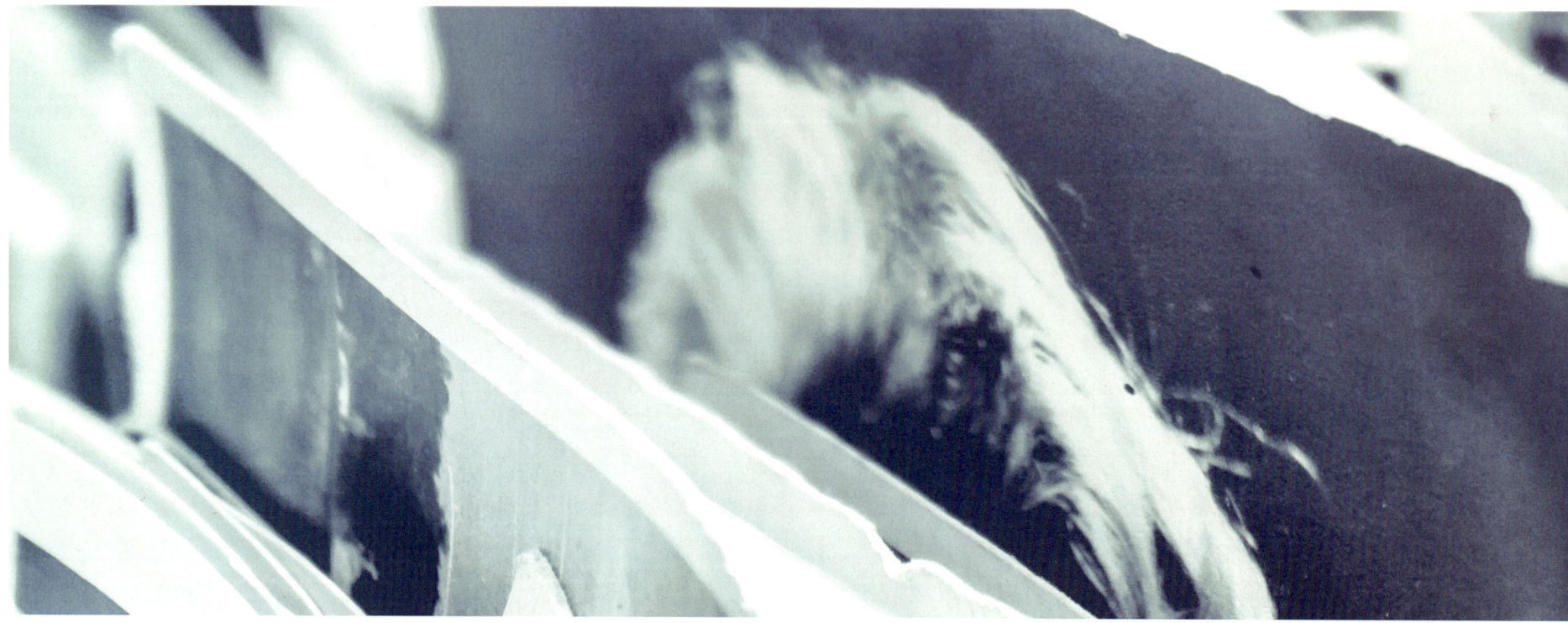

It is also important to note that Mikao Usui did not base his Reiki practice on the chakra system. Like all other therapeutic practices from East Asia, older Reiki therapies use the meridian system. However, newer Reiki modalities often incorporate the chakras because their ethos fits very well with Reiki practices.

And although Reiki was developed with the meridian system in mind rather than the chakra system, it is perfectly valid to suggest that Reiki (and the other facets of Ki) interacts with the chakras. Reiki powers the human energy system and chakras are one way of expressing that system, even though they are derived from different cultural perspectives.

Now, whilst it is vital for you to form your own perspective about the chakra system, it does help to have a foundation to work from. So here is a very basic, quick reference list of the chakras and some associated beliefs.

A chakra may be seen as *open*—spinning in a balanced fashion—or as *closed*—spinning sluggishly, spinning too fast, rotating the wrong way, etc.

When the chakras are closed:

- Base Chakra closed: Emotionally needy, low self-esteem, self-destructive behaviour, fearful.

- Sacral Chakra closed: Oversensitive, hard on him/her/zirself, feels guilty for no reason, low libido or sexual dysfunction.

- Solar Plexus Chakra closed: Overly concerned with what others think, fearful of being alone, insecure, needs constant reassurance.

- Heart Chakra closed: Fears rejection, loves too much, feels unworthy to receive love, self-pitying.

- Throat Chakra closed: Holds back from self-expression, unreliable. Holds inconsistent views.

- Third Eye Chakra closed: Undisciplined, fears success, tendency towards schizophrenia, sets sights too low.

- Crown Chakra closed: Constantly exhausted, cannot make decisions, no sense of *belonging*.

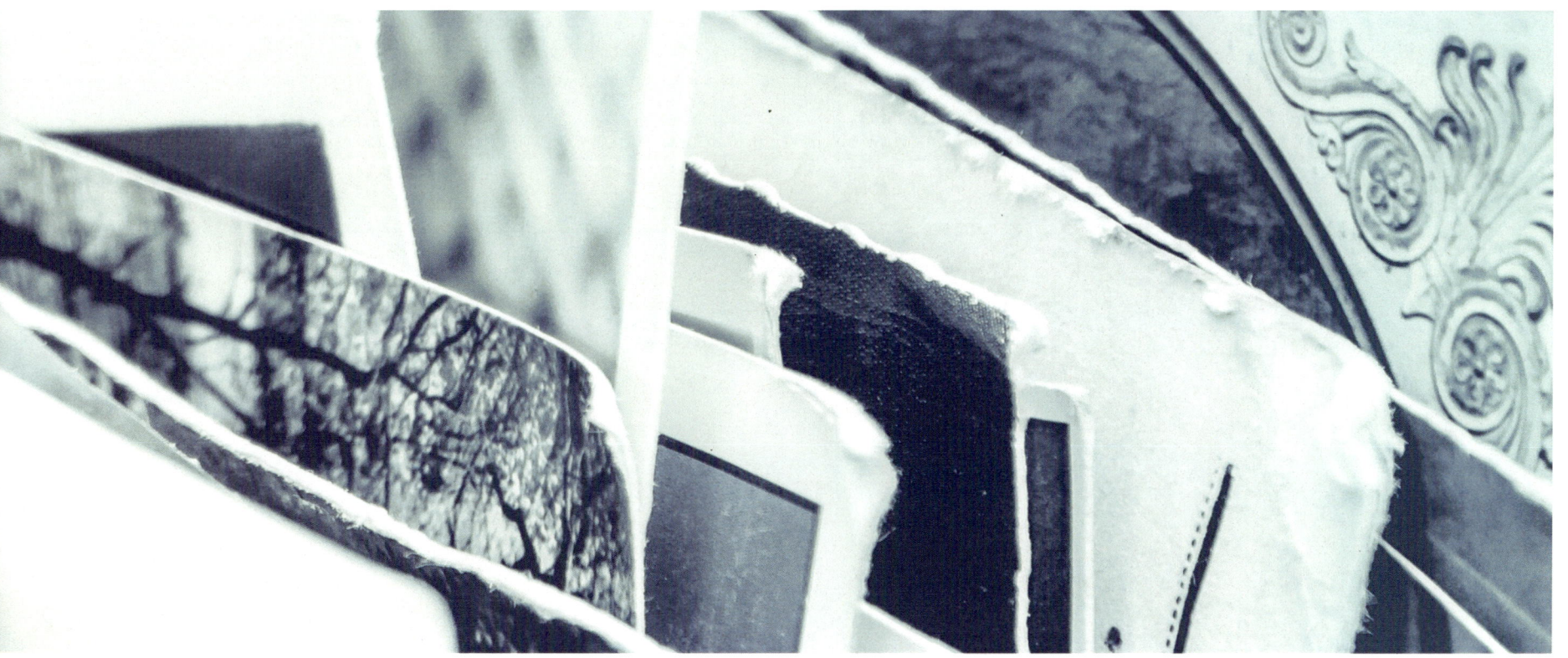

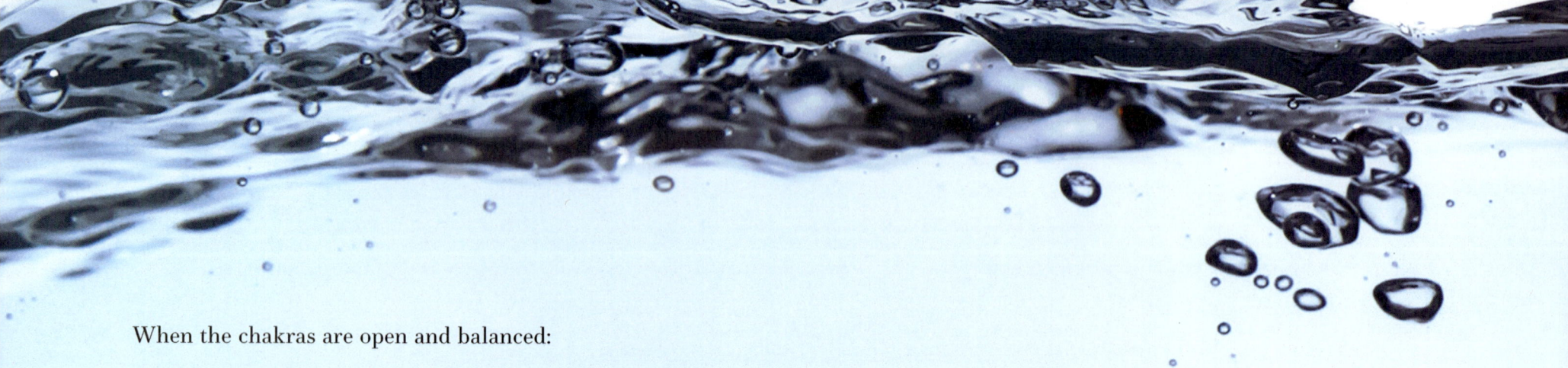

When the chakras are open and balanced:

- Base Chakra open: Demonstrates self-mastery, high physical energy, grounded, healthy.
- Sacral Chakra open: Trusting, expressive, attuned to his/her/zir own feelings, creative.
- Solar Plexus Chakra open: Respects self and others, has personal power, spontaneous, uninhibited.
- Heart Chakra open: Compassionate, loves unconditionally, nurturing, desires spiritual experience in lovemaking:
- Throat Chakra open: Good communicator, contented, finds it easy to meditate, artistically inspired.
- Third Eye Chakra open: Charismatic, highly intuitive, not attached to material things, may experience unusual phenomena.
- Crown Chakra open: Magnetic personality, achieves *miracles* in life, transcendent, at peace with self.

When the chakras are spinning too fast:

- Base Chakra spinning too fast: Bullying, overly materialistic, self-centred, engages in physical foolhardiness.
- Sacral Chakra spinning too fast: Emotionally unbalanced, a fantasist, manipulative, sexually addictive.
- Solar Plexus Chakra spinning too fast: Angry, controlling, workaholic, judgemental and superior.
- Heart Chakra spinning too fast: Possessive, loves conditionally, withholds emotionally to *punish*, overly dramatic.
- Throat Chakra spinning too fast: Over-talkative, dogmatic, self-righteous, arrogant.
- Third Eye Chakra spinning too fast: Highly logical, dogmatic, authoritarian, arrogant.
- Crown Chakra spinning too fast: Psychotic or manic depressive, confused sexual expression, frustrated, sense of unrealised power.

The Eastern knowledge of physiology and therapy was developed over millennia, with practitioners, academics, teachers, masters and gurus matching the symptoms of their clients with their own intuitive and sensory experiences. Over time, these elaborate observation records evolved into the therapies and methods we know today.

The Western approach to physiology and medicine is very different; we cut people open and record what we see. This may be an actual visual observation or a more indirect scientific observation using equipment, tests, etc.

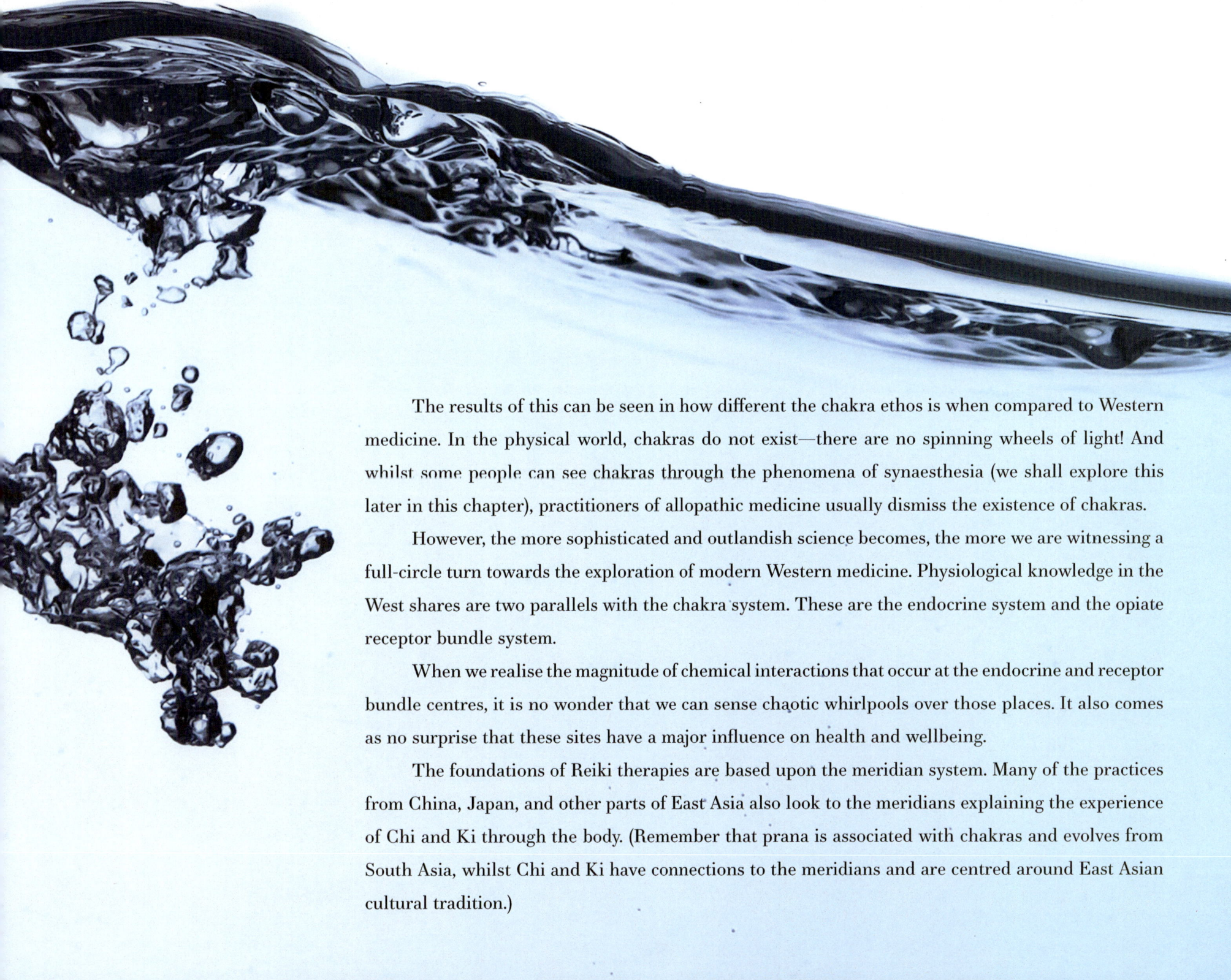

The results of this can be seen in how different the chakra ethos is when compared to Western medicine. In the physical world, chakras do not exist—there are no spinning wheels of light! And whilst some people can see chakras through the phenomena of synaesthesia (we shall explore this later in this chapter), practitioners of allopathic medicine usually dismiss the existence of chakras.

However, the more sophisticated and outlandish science becomes, the more we are witnessing a full-circle turn towards the exploration of modern Western medicine. Physiological knowledge in the West shares are two parallels with the chakra system. These are the endocrine system and the opiate receptor bundle system.

When we realise the magnitude of chemical interactions that occur at the endocrine and receptor bundle centres, it is no wonder that we can sense chaotic whirlpools over those places. It also comes as no surprise that these sites have a major influence on health and wellbeing.

The foundations of Reiki therapies are based upon the meridian system. Many of the practices from China, Japan, and other parts of East Asia also look to the meridians explaining the experience of Chi and Ki through the body. (Remember that prana is associated with chakras and evolves from South Asia, whilst Chi and Ki have connections to the meridians and are centred around East Asian cultural tradition.)

In Eastern medicine, there are a dozen pairs of meridians that extend along the length of the body. In addition to these twelve pairs of meridians, there are two additional meridians: one traversing the front of the body from perineum to head, and the other travelling along the spine, from perineum to head. These midline meridians are known as the *conception* and *governing* vessels.

In traditions originating in China, Chi is seen to flow through these channels, creating a complex dynamic throughout the body. In Japan, the philosophy uses an exact model of the meridians, but changes the force, or Universal Constant, to Ki.

When treating a client, the practitioner seeks to determine a good flow of Chi or Ki through each meridian; noticing when meridians are blocked or the Chi/Ki flow is either too strong or too weak. A meridian-based practitioner will take six pulses on each wrist to determine which meridian is blocked and how the Chi/Ki is flowing through the system.

It is important to note that, once again, meridians are not recognised in modern Western medicine. However, modern science has identified a living matrix of systems within the body that mirrors the ethos of meridians.

Our nerves, blood vessels, skeletal structure, and muscles are coated with a liquid crystal structure that vibrates messages across the body. This crystalline coating, along with the skin and the digestive system, forms a living matrix that communicates and coordinates our bodies' natural healing functions.

Whenever a person experiences some form of dis-ease, injury or dysfunction, this is reflected in the vibrations flowing through the living matrix. The body responds by sending healing agents to the site of injury, infection, etc. However, the living matrix also communicates an infinite array of vibrational, analogue information.

The vibrations that permeate the living matrix, regardless of the specific frequency, contain energy. They have their own force and, therefore, could be viewed as analogous to the meridians. Whenever we alter the vibrations through the living matrix, regardless of this alteration being initiated internally or externally (from the environment) the changes will affect the whole person, what they feel, and how they heal.

Our final area of physiology is, perhaps, the most enigmatic and hotly debated. The aura or auric field is the most important system we encounter in Karmic Reiki, because although we work with the meridians and chakras, it is in the aura that regression is experienced. Additionally, in the layers of the auric field we establish what challenges our clients face and how to heal them.

Indeed, in the original form of Karmic Reiki, the method was also known as Auric Reiki; an indication of how invested we are in the treatment of the aura.

If the meridians govern the experience of energy in the physical body and the chakras are transmission gateways between the body and the outside world, the aura is an extension of the physical body that extends into the physical environment and beyond.

The vibrations of all physical, emotional, mental and spiritual functions resonate within and around the physical body, forming layers—like a vibrational onion skin! This is due to the variation of frequency and amplitude of the different vibrations; which we can understand as similar to the effect of mixing oil and water.

The denser vibrations (higher frequency and amplitude) exist closest to the physical body (the densest auric layer of all). Conversely, vibrations become less dense (lower in frequency and/or amplitude) as our focus moves outward.

Whilst we refer to layers in the auric field, each section does not actually finish where another begins—the aura is rather like a spectrum of vibrations. The vibrations naturally pool in certain areas, creating distinct layers. However, these layers do extend into each other in one connected and holistic entity.

There are four main layers, or *bodies*, in the auric field: The *etheric*, the *emotional*, the *psychological* and the *spiritual*.

The etheric body carries a vibrational blueprint of the physical body, governing how physically healthy a person is. Traditionally, it is believed that a system of channels known as *nadis*, extends throughout the etheric body. The vibrancy and overall health of these vibrational channels determine the health of the person.

Certain types of vibrations filtering through from other levels of the aura or the external environment can disrupt the healthy state of the nadis; causing blocks and eventually dis-ease.

The emotional body is reflected in our emotional health, our feelings, and our desires. A healthy auric layer will manifest health in a person's emotional state. Yet, the emotional health of a person is also reflected in changes to the emotional body of the aura.

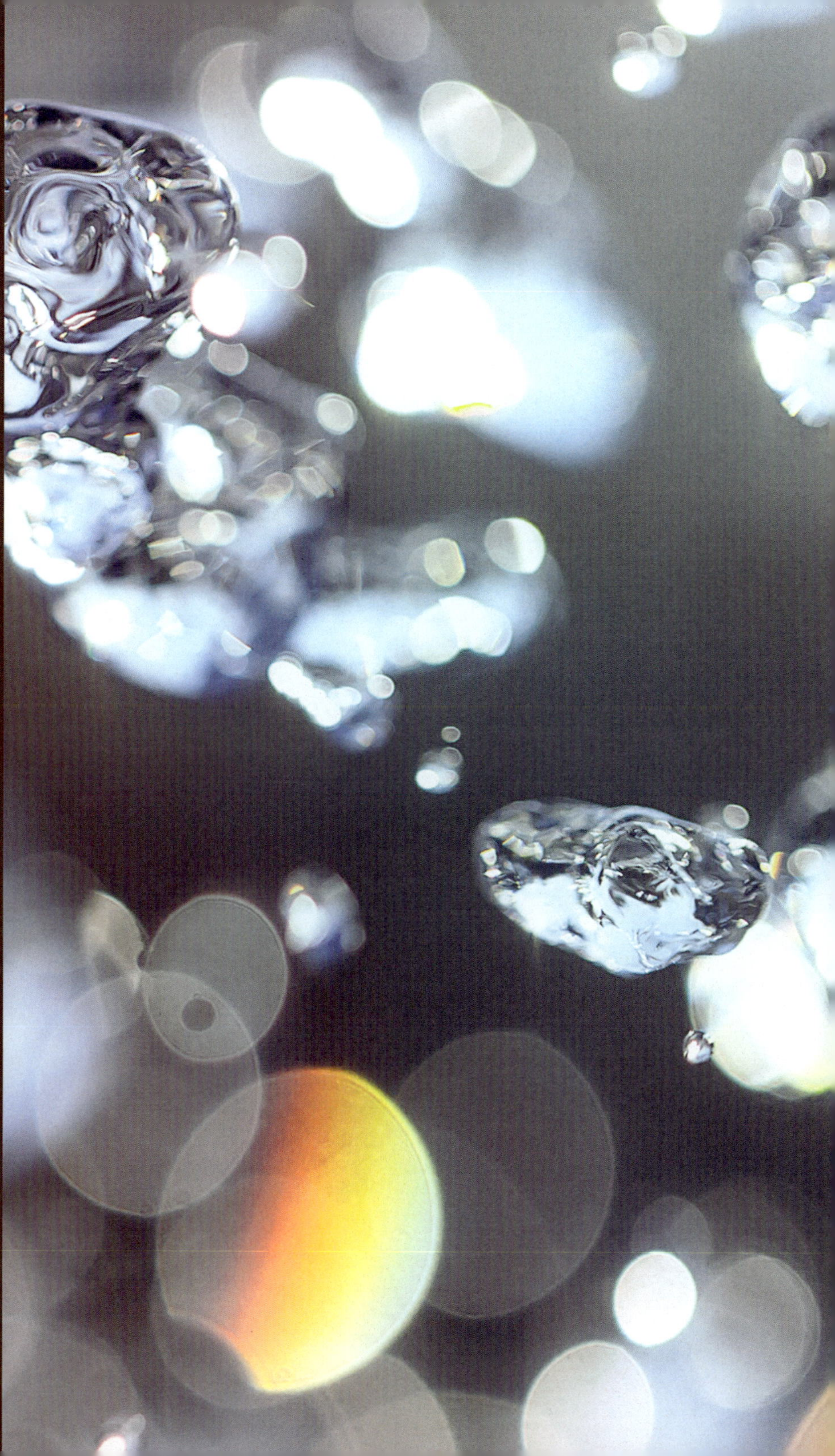

The psychological body is where our thoughts are both mirrored and seeded. This layer is not where we usually think it is (inside our brain and nervous system). Thought patterns created in the brain are influenced by the mental body and these, in turn, influence this layer of the aura. The healthier the vibrational state, the healthier the thoughts we think, and vice versa!

Lastly, we encounter the spiritual body, where the blueprint for our inner wisdom, or *Higher Self,* is said to reside. This auric layer relates to our spiritual growth and how we progress along our path. Although we are affected by *who we were born to be*, what really counts is how we act on a daily basis and how this relates to our life purpose.

The spiritual body consists of various sub-layers. One of which is often referred to as the *causal body*. The causal body reflects our actions and inherent nature—everything we came into the world with and what many would view as our *soul* is enveloped in this level.

In modern terms, our understanding of the auric field can grow in complexity and become overwhelming very quickly. From the vibrations all around us, to quantum theory, the ideas and attitudes of our society/community and the emotions of those around us. We could view the aura as the transmission layer between us and the physical/etheric environment around us.

As we navigate through the world and etheric environments we come into contact with, the experiences affect us profoundly, regardless of our being consciously aware of those experiences or not. We have various mechanisms that filter, generalise, delete and distort what we sense, experience and understand from without.

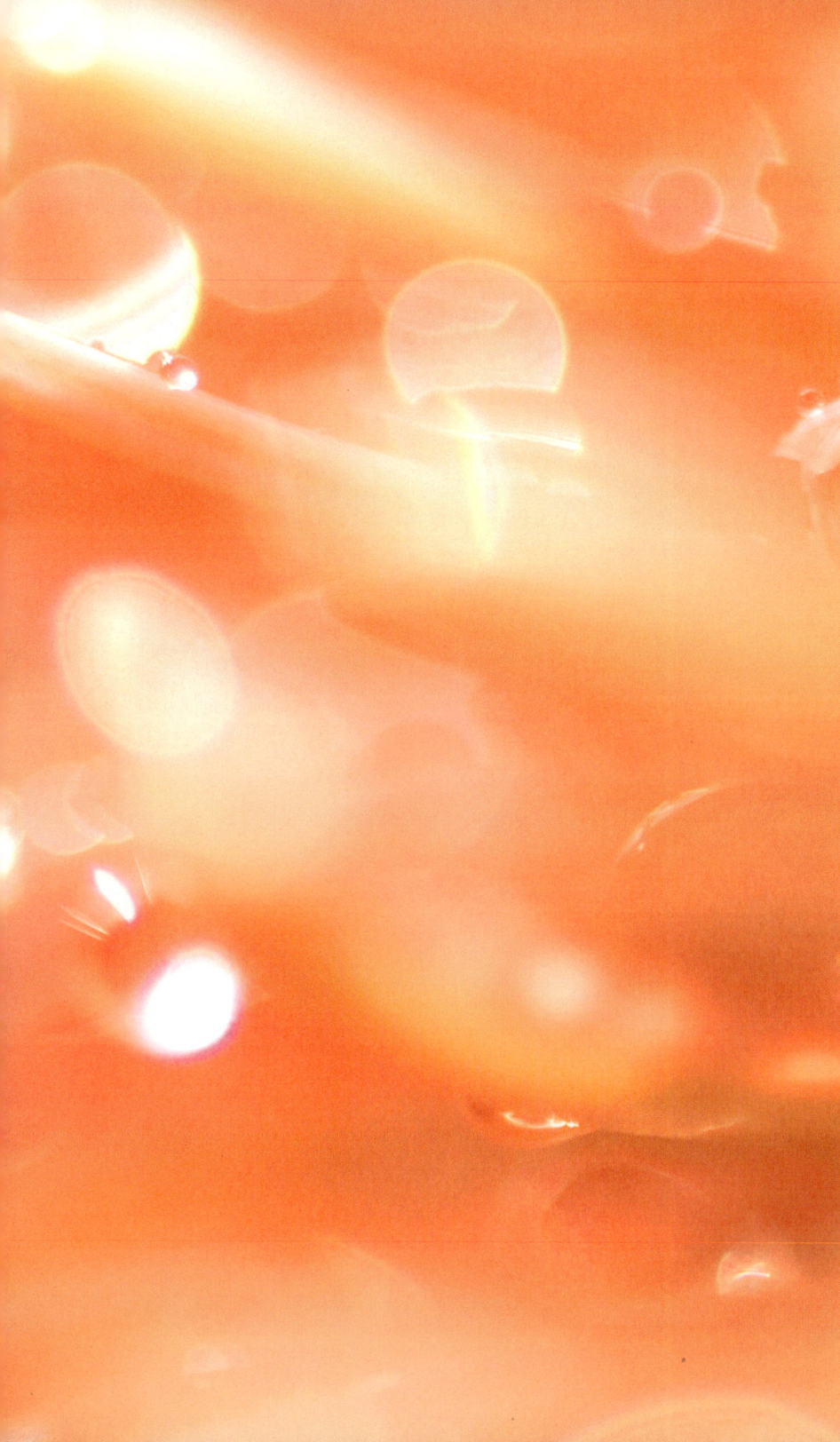

These mechanisms act as gatekeepers to what exists for us in potential and what we perceive in reality.

This does not mean these gatekeepers guard us against detrimental experiences. What they do is affect to what we pay attention, how we experience life, and the level of health/wellbeing we enjoy. As we are immersed in the stimuli bombarding us from the outside world, our senses recognise different aspects of this stimuli.

We see things, hear things, feel things, taste, and smell things. We also experience synaesthesia, another important aspect of Karmic Reiki and KRT. As a practitioner of KRT, you will need to recognise and identify your own synaesthesia to interpret treatments for your clients.

Synaesthesia comes in many forms and is basically a way in which your brain processes information that it cannot understand or that extends to a level of detail beyond the usual degree of sensory awareness. One of the most common forms of synaesthesia is feeling physical pain when we see somebody else being injured. This is similar to feeling an emotional response to another person's pain.

Most empaths and sympaths experience varying degrees of synaesthesia, although the particular type of synaesthesia you experience and how profound that is, will depend on your unique perspective.

Some people see flashes of colour or complex shapes when hearing sounds, other hear sounds when touching objects or people. There are those who experience colours as different tastes or smell different aromas when reading words. The forms of

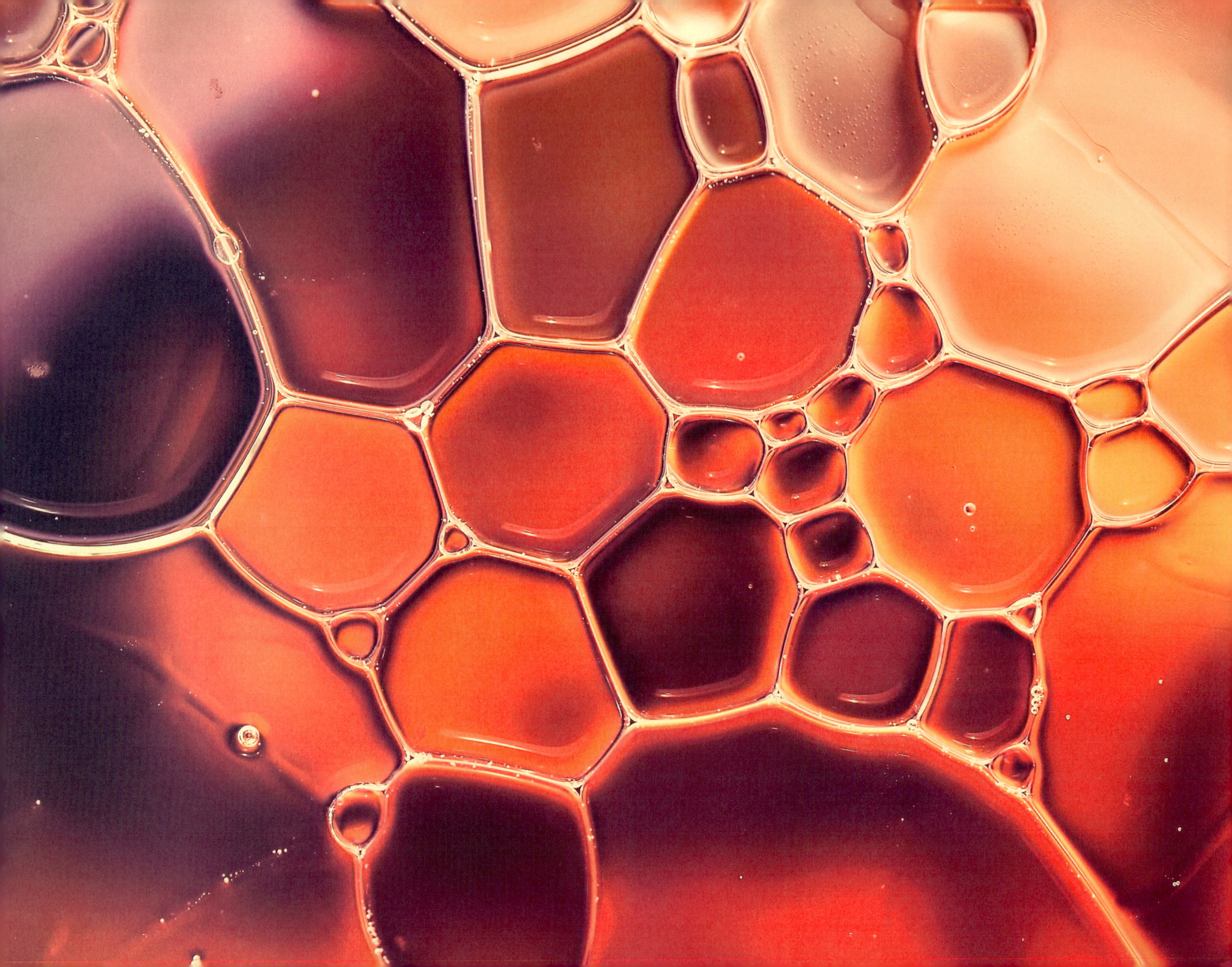

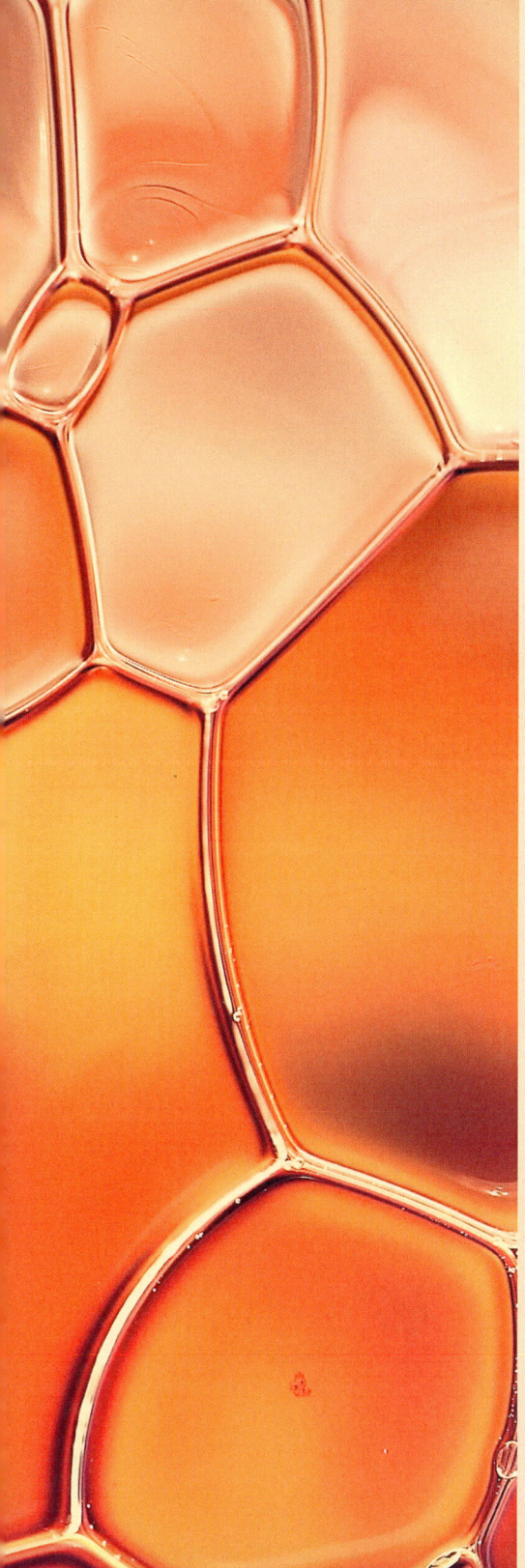
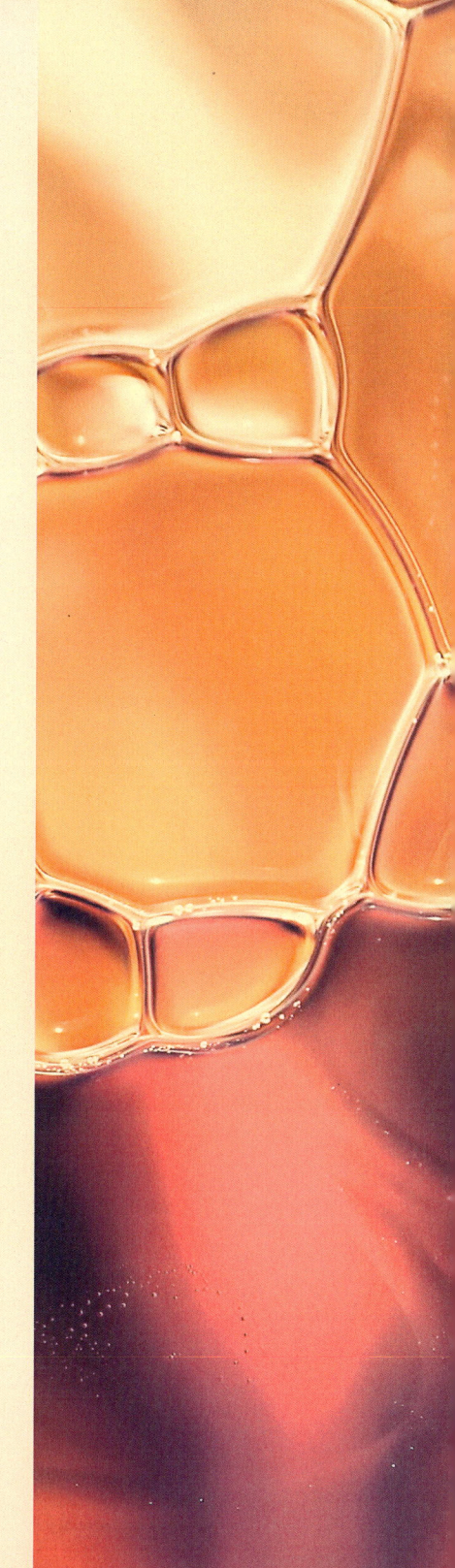

synaesthesia we are most focused on in KRT are the sensory feedback experiences gained from our living matrix vibrations.

As you work within the vibrations of your client's auric field, you will use your synaesthetic abilities to feel, see, hear, feel, taste, and smell reactions to the different frequencies and amplitudes you perceive. These sensations will form the basis of your interpretations and client feedback.

Whilst you are interpreting the experiences synaesthetically during a treatment, you may find your client also manifests synaesthetic sensory experiences that will add clarity to your feedback. However, there are occasions when you and your client will experience very different aspects of the same treatment.

This is not because you are doing anything *wrong*, or even because you are recognising different things. It is simply that everybody is uniquely different and experiences the world in different and even contrasting ways.

Once you have calibrated to your perspective of Karmic Reiki, practised the basic treatment methods of Reiji Ho and Byosen Reikan Ho, and understood the foundational physiology of our therapy—including the concept of synaesthesia—you will be ready to start working with Karmic Reiki and Karmic Regression Therapy. In the next chapter, we will step into the realm of regression and discover what awaits for us in the Karmic State.

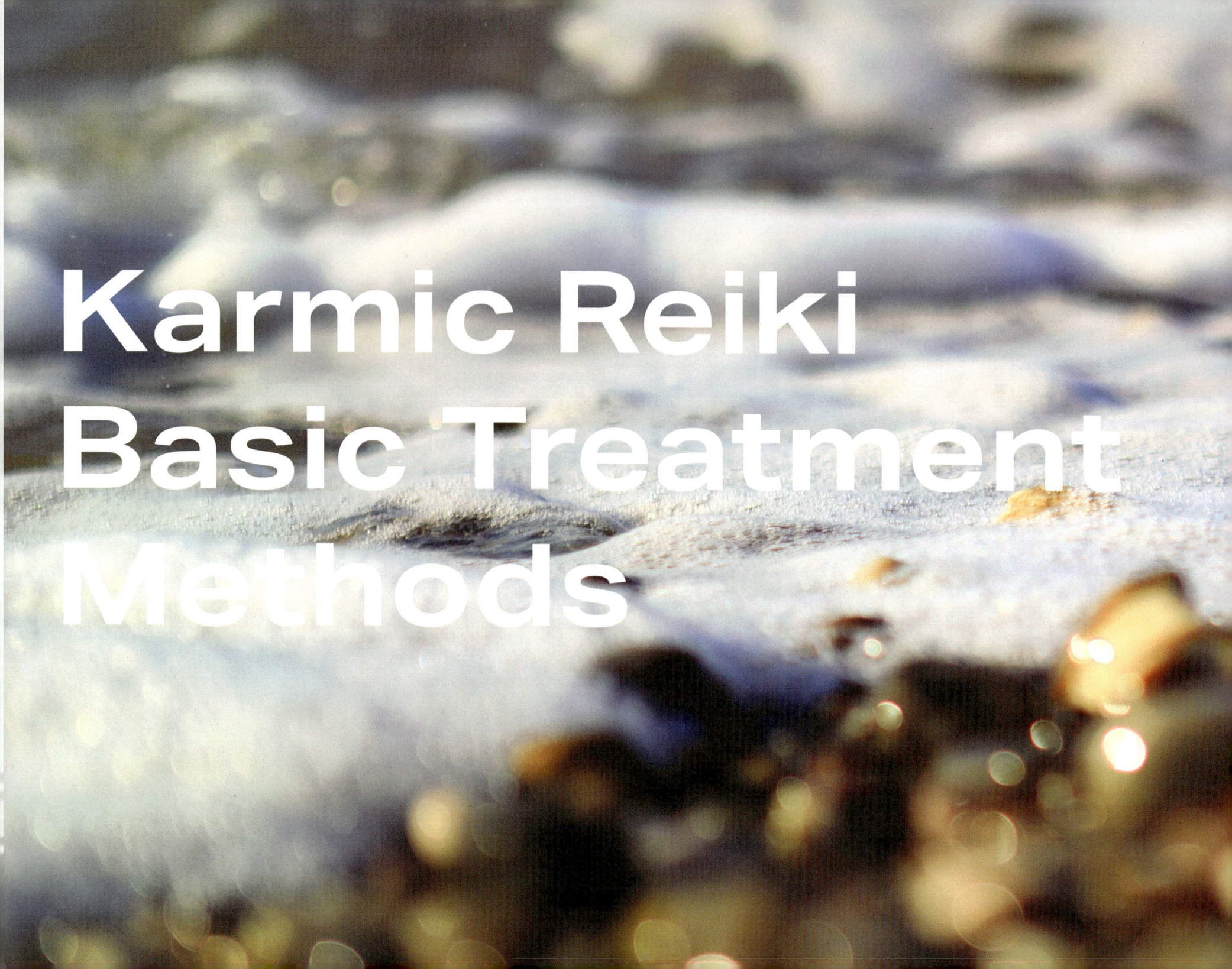

Karmic Reiki Basic Treatment Methods

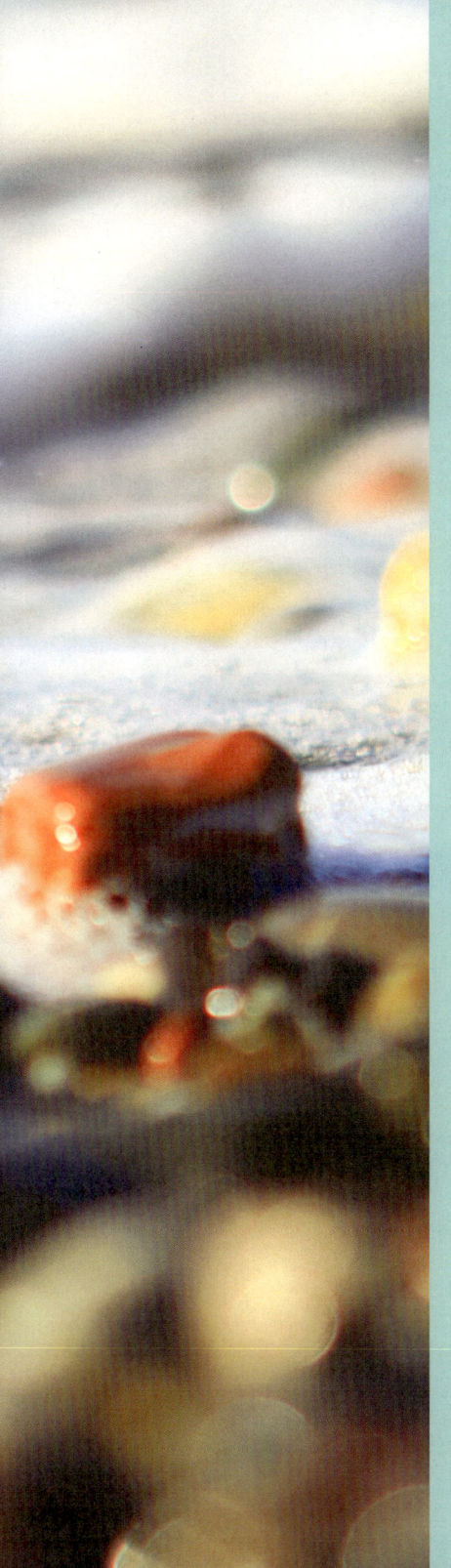

While there are **five different layers** in our Karmic Regression Therapy Practice, from Karmic Reiki to vKRT, there are only three treatment styles.

You are only likely to use the second or third of these styles with any regularity. Despite this, the first treatment method is included here for historical context and also as a step on your learning path.

The important (and regularly used) tools of treatment involve The Karmic Sisters in Karmic Reiki and the Box Treatments of KRT. Yet, we will begin with a miscellaneous collection of treatment styles that will enable to you create a very basic form of treatment using contrasting experiences of Reiki. These are based on the westernised versions of Usui Reiki and, if you are familiar with Usui Reiki or Usui Teate, will find an easy segue into Karmic Reiki.

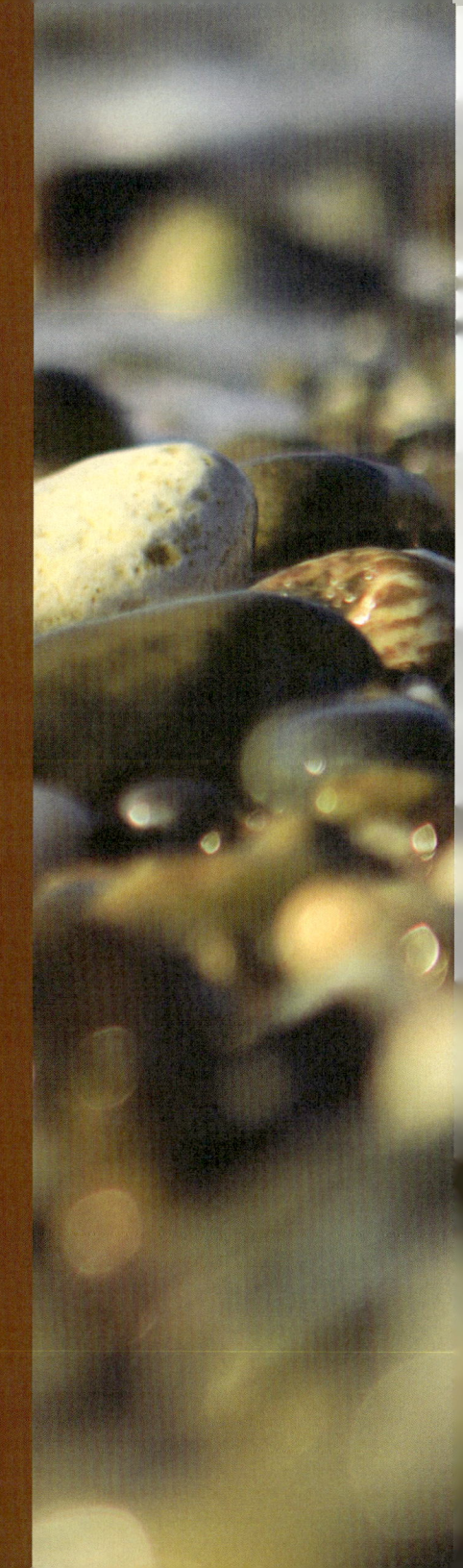

In the practice of Usui Reiki therapies, professional therapists will often use symbolic triggers to alter their experience of the force driving the treatment. Some westernised versions of Reiki modalities include non-traditional symbols, triggering bespoke healing perspectives.

It was whilst using these different perspectives (and their associated symbols) that I began to recognise the initial effects of a Karmic State: icy cold environment and an ominous sensation of darkness! To help introduce you to the Karmic State, here is a selection of Reiki modality symbols that directly affect the Karmic State and can initiate a regression experience.

These are not KRT-based experiences, which are very different. However, they do offer an idea of what to expect at first, whilst easing yourself into the very dramatic effects of Karmic Reiki and KRT.

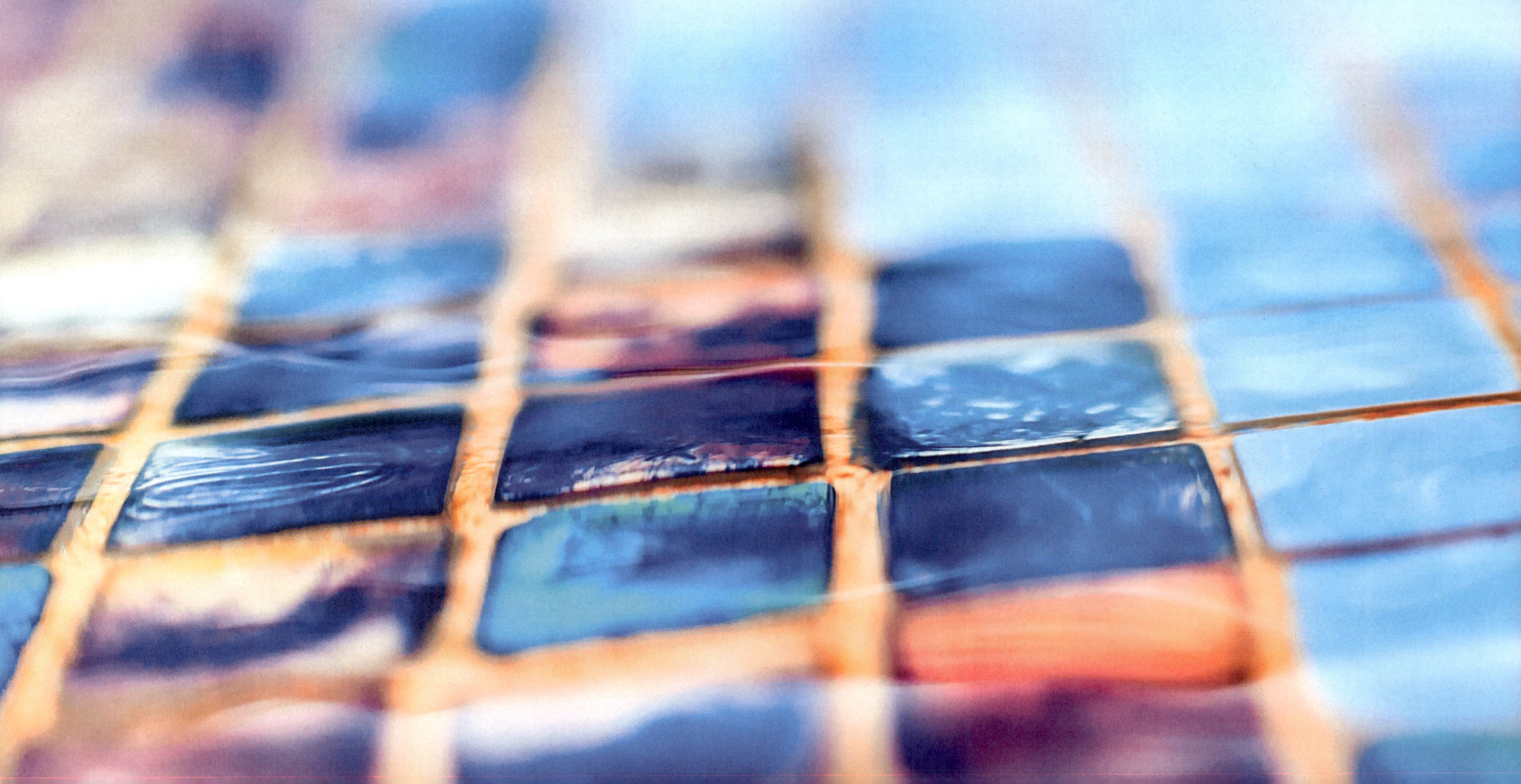

Taoist Grace

Grace works to clear repetitive or habitual behaviour created by karmic issues, including contractive thought patterns and birth trauma. When vibrations create a contractive response in your client, Grace can be applied to neutralise the reaction in conjunction with the client working on the underlying cause.

For example, with karmic overeating—if the client works with the root cause of the overeating, the Taoist Grace symbol can be used to clear any damage done. It may be that the client has dismissed the root cause already and that only the karmic treatment is required.

To use Grace, draw it over the whole body or on your hands and then use in the psychological body of the aura.

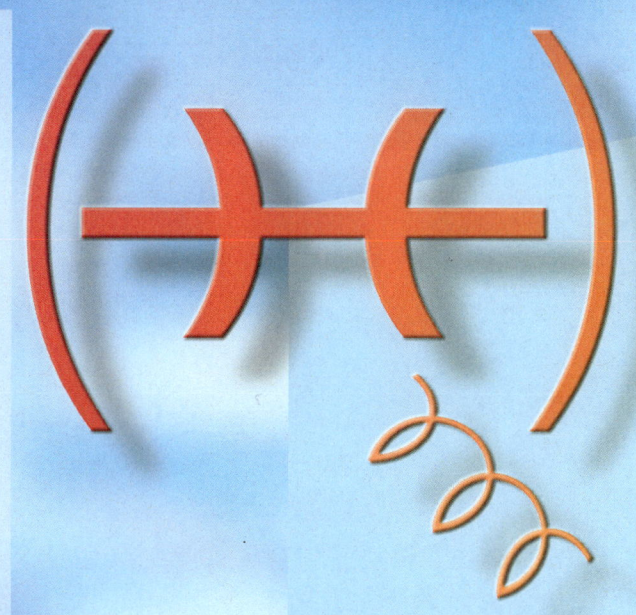

The Emotional Butterfly— Karmic Cleanser

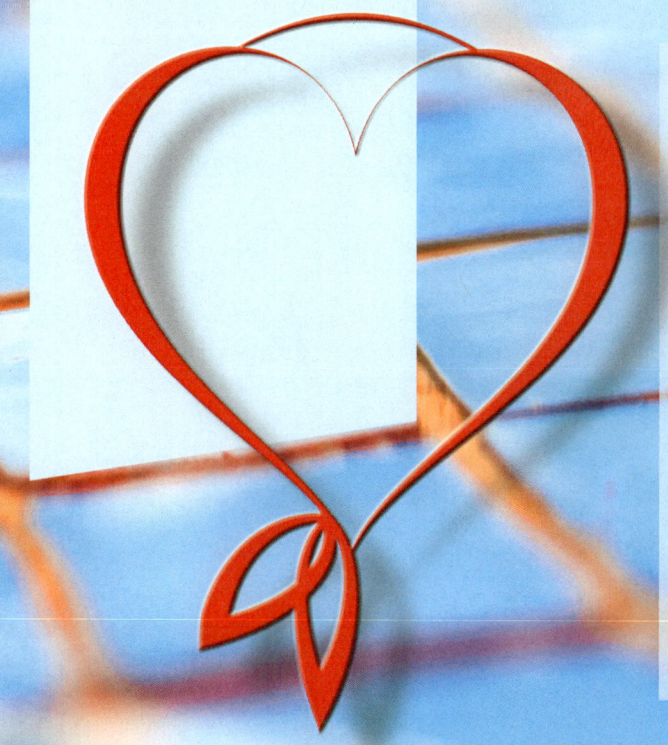

This perspective of Reiki applies to the emotional side of karmic issues, bringing subconscious emotional patterns and habits into the conscious mind so the client can deal with them. It can be used in conjunction with the Grace perspective and is often followed by Grace in a karmic treatment.

Again, the symbol can be visualised over the entire body, drawn on hands and placed in the emotional body or drawn over the heart chakra.

Contraindications: It can cause emotional release. Remember to advise clients of this effect and the possible detoxification process that can follow a treatment.

Beyond Usui Reiki, there are various Karmic-related perspectives from other modalities. Here are some examples that you may wish to work with.

Zonar (Zoe-nar)

Zonar means *infinity* or *eternity* and is thought to work with karmic patterns stored at a cellular level. Working in conjunction with the next perspective (Halu), Zonar can be applied as a preparation for the deeper, more intense experiences triggered by Halu.

Zonar is applied to help us work through past issues, birth trauma and child abuse, whether they are conscious, or subconscious memories. Zonar can bring about conscious awareness of lessons that need to be learnt or situations that, when healed, will negate karmic patterns—this eliminates the need to work directly with a karmic issue that can sometimes be too painful and traumatic for the subject.

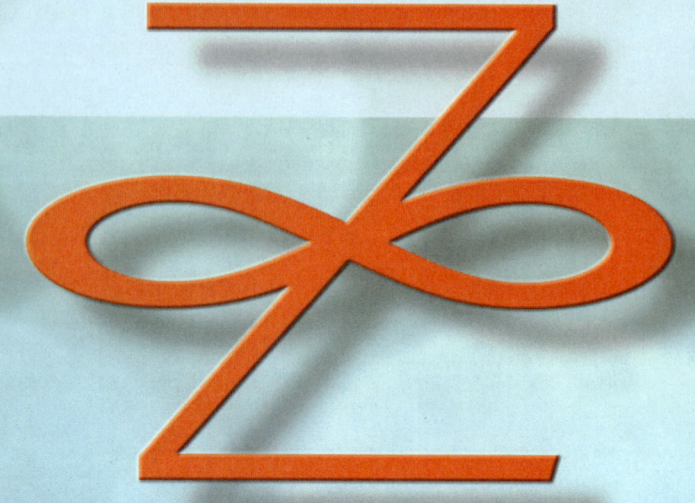

Halu (Hay-Loo)

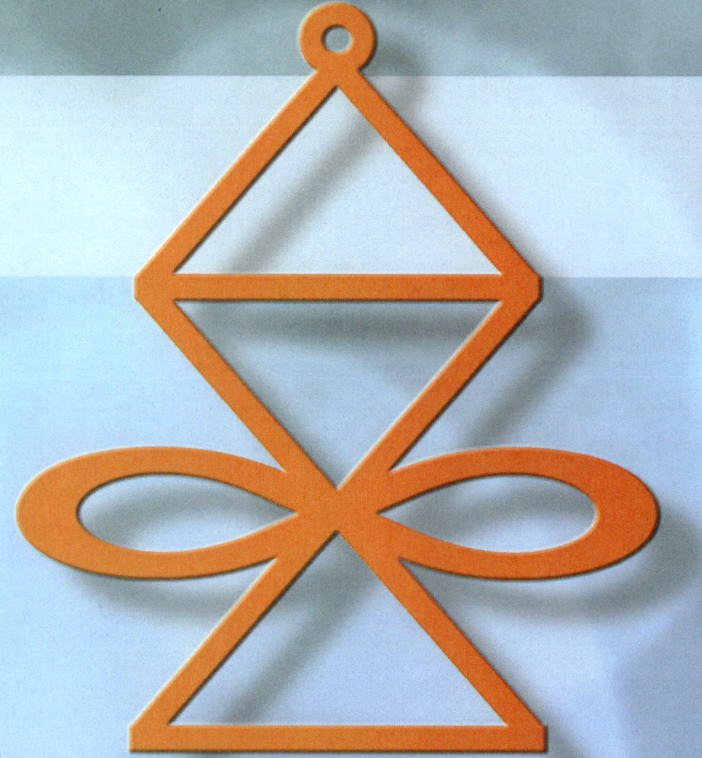

Halu means *truth* and is seen as an amplification of Zonar, working in higher levels of consciousness and at deeper levels of subconscious experience. Used directly after the first perspective of Zonar, Halu restores balance and is thought to bring about *deep healing* at the causal and karmic layers of the auric field.

Similar to the emotional/psychological perspective of Usui Reiki Therapy, Halu assists in the dissolution of contractive karmic patterns in the subconscious mind—those that keep us from the truth—and overthrows both delusion and denial.

Halu is a wonderful tool for breaking down the illusions given to us by society, such as limiting beliefs, social programming or pigeonholing, etc. It is also used to open experiences of higher consciousness.

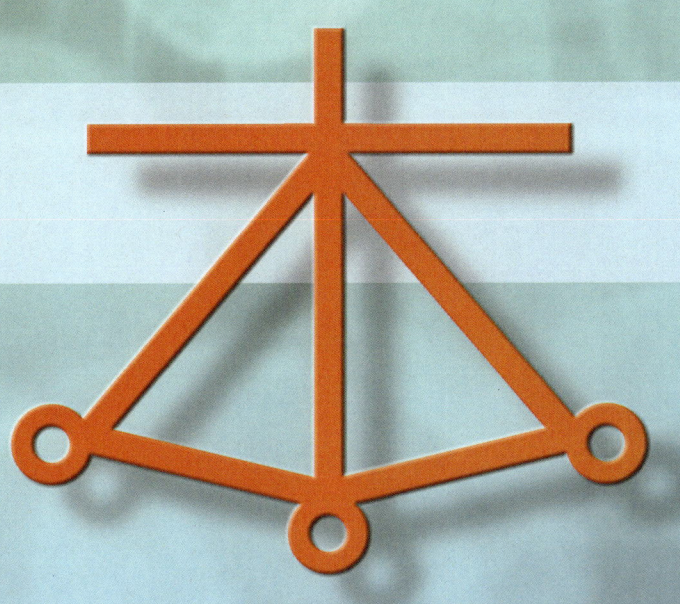

Harth

Harth embodies an all-encompassing love, representing the infinite love and compassion of the universe. Revolving around the ability to empathise with the pain and trauma of others, Harth allows each of us to break down the illusion of powerlessness—of feeling unable to help. This stops us from standing idly by when others need help, empowering us to make a difference.

Harth envelops us with the strength of universal benevolence; guiding and supporting us, healing the heart and helping one develop compassion for others. Useful when healing relationships, Harth restores our love of life and each other.

In terms of karmic patterns, Harth has a profound effect when treating addictions of all kinds. The powerful treatment offered by Harth melts away the core traumas and challenges that are fertile ground for addictive habits.

Rama

Rama translates into joy. The perspective here opens, connects, and balances the lower chakras to the earth, then aligns the upper chakras with the lower. When applied in treatment, Rama works very well with all issues pertaining to problematic functions of the lower chakras such as power struggles, grounding, sexual issues, body function, and image.

The results with the lower chakras, along with the alignment of the higher centres means that Rama works very well with the concept of manifestation and goal realisation. If you work with the Foot chakras from this perspective along with the power symbol of Usui Reiki, the combined effort will connect the feet to the Earth—bringing balance and increasing the connection to Ki.

The impact of Rama on chakra alignment makes it a powerful karmic harmoniser—balancing and syncing all chakras to a common rhythm.

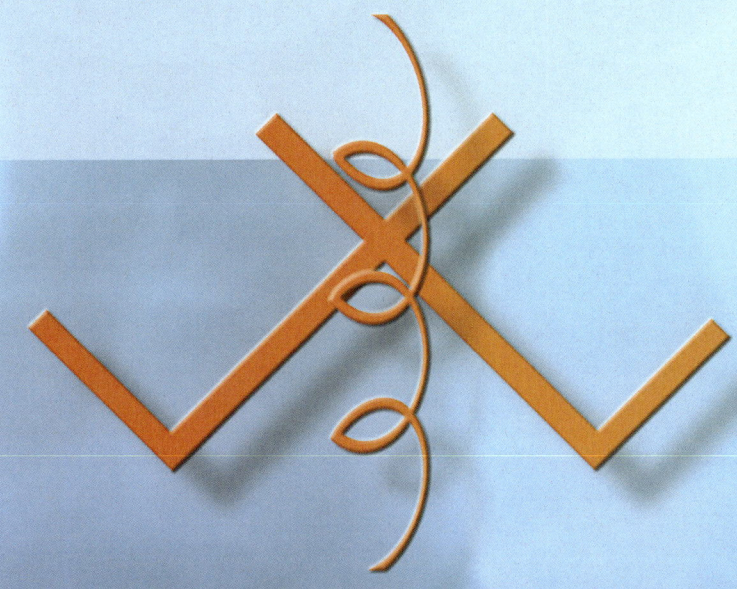

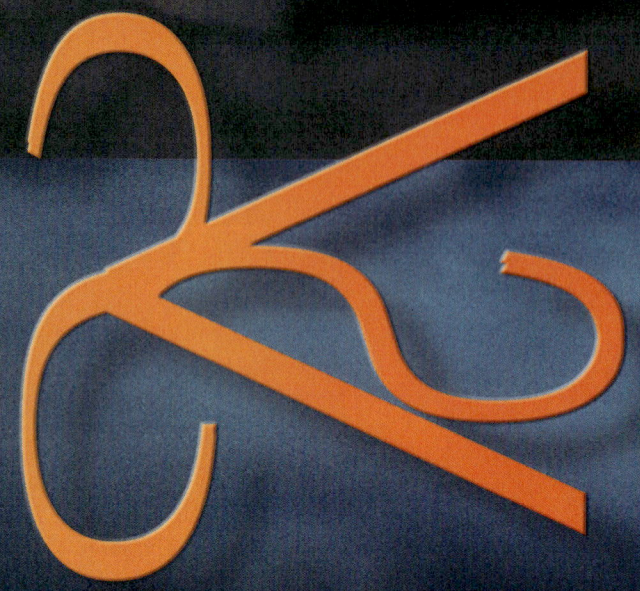

Shanti (Shawn-Tee)

Shanti, *peace*, supports the healing of past hurts and traumas, so we may live freely in the present moment—unfettered by the traumas and memories that often hold us back. Holding on to past situations and obsolete dreams keeps us from investing time into a better future—one that is appropriate for our life purpose. Shanti can help us to release outdated perspectives to create a better future vision.

Shanti can be applied to break karmic patterns—those we repeat because of past trauma or dis-ease. This not only allows us to find new paths, but also helps us become unstuck from the aspects of life that keep us bound in repeating cycles.

Dumo (Dum-moe)

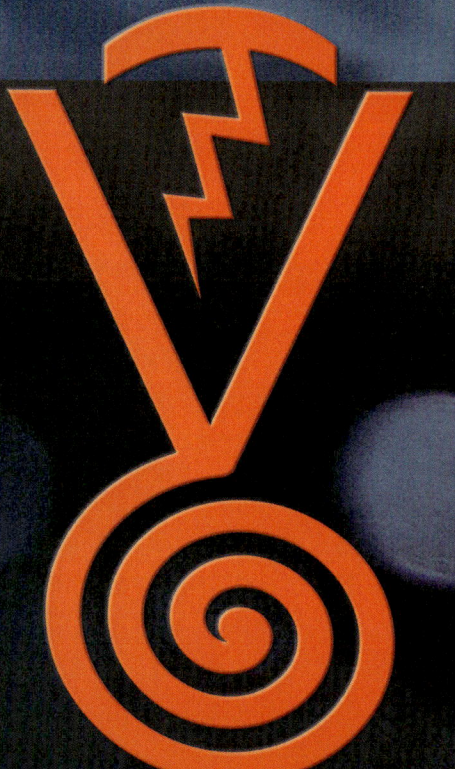

The symbolic representation of the Dumo perspective represents a goblet or receptacle being cleansed by a lightning bolt—and that is the main application of this experience in a therapeutic sense.

Whilst not as strong as the Usui Reiki Master Perspective, the Tibetan version is a cleanser used to replenish the chakra system in preparation for traditional attunement methods. Dumo can also be applied to treatments where deep karmic cleansing is needed.

Application of a Foundation Karmic Experience

Before exploring the methodology of Karmic Reiki, we can combine both Reijo Ho and Byosen Reikan Ho treatments with the above perspectives of Reiki therapies. Beginning with scanning for byosen and triggering the preferred perspective when cleansing hibiki, the practitioner can then transition to Reiji Ho and combine this free-flow practice with other perspectives.

For example, as you are simply letting the treatment take place, you might add Taoist Grace to enhance the effect on your client. At any point in the session, if your hands move to the heart area, you can apply The Emotional Butterfly or perhaps Harth.

You could apply Dumo at the beginning of the treatment, work through the series of Zonar, Halu Harth, and Rama, or perhaps apply Shanti when you encounter obstacles to treatment. Each of the perspectives triggered by the symbols above, can be brought to treatment as you intuit—depending on how you feel and what you believe to be appropriate at that time for your client.

Certainly, working with these traditional techniques and the addition of the karmic perspectives of Reiki during the early days of training and practice, will help prepare you for the Karmic Reiki experience. However, this treatment combination is also useful when treating clients professionally.

At times and for a multitude of reasons, you may not experience any discernible results during treatment; if this is the case, know that these traditional treatment styles offer a means of treating your client in an extremely impactful way, without the intuitive and interpretive feedback of Karmic Reiki.

As you progress into the more advanced iterations of KRT practice, you will come to realise that what you do with your hands and how you treat your client in the physical environment is less important than what is happening beyond the physical experience.

In these circumstances, you may choose to initiate treatment and then use the traditional treatment discussed here to provide a dual treatment for your client. In this way, the forty-five-minute treatment will contain both a traditional treatment and a powerful KRT treatment, whilst giving you something practical to do and demonstrating to your client that you are not simply sitting in the corner twiddling your thumbs!

Of course, in this scenario, you may have other forms of therapy to conduct after initiating the KRT treatment, such as massage or other therapy modality. Whichever treatment style you decide to use, the traditional methods here will help you hone your professional skills as a Karmic Regression therapist.

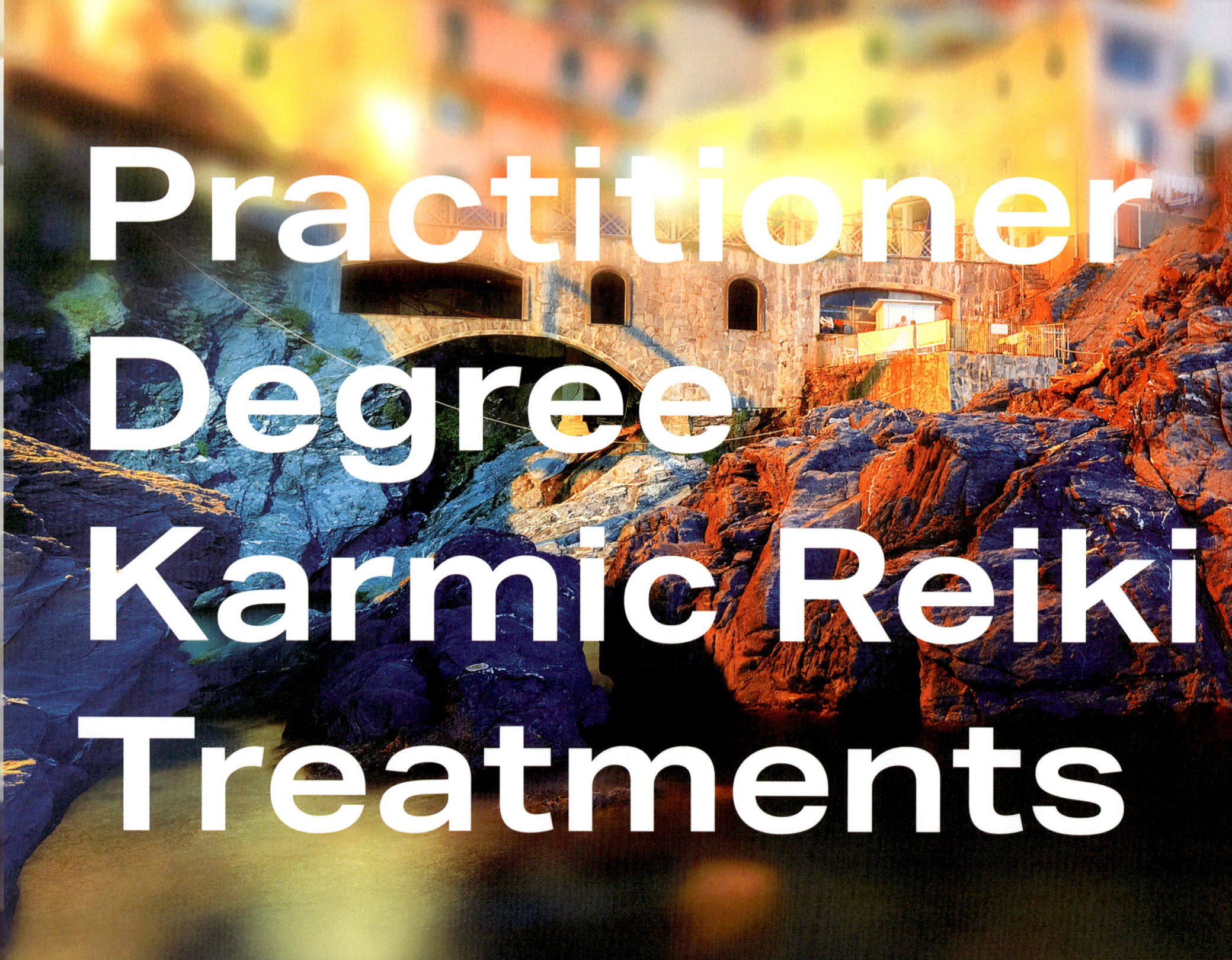

Practitioner Degree Karmic Reiki Treatments

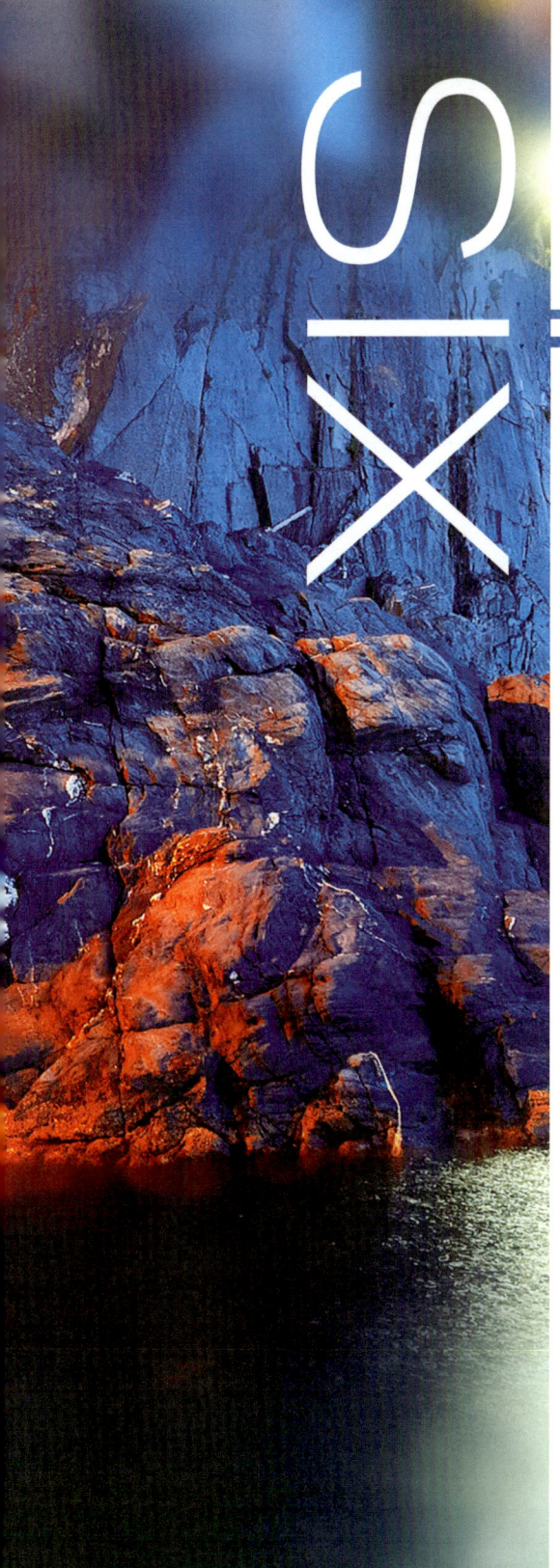

Once you have developed a confident approach to the foundations of Karmic Reiki, it is time to progress to the professional, practitioner degree of treatment. Here, you are not only following a more formal style of treatment but also using your intuitive and synaesthetic abilities to interpret feedback for your client.

The treatment style itself is very simple to work. Similar to both Byosen Reikan Ho and Reiji Ho combined, it is a series of steps that open up a vast world of experiences. Using three perspectives of Karmic Reiki, you enter a Karmic State with your client, you then sense, intuit, and interpret the different forms that are experienced.

These many karmic objects, karmic events or other subtle experiences tend to reveal themselves in Karmic Reiki treatments. Once these have been noted, understood, and possibly elaborated upon, you vaporise these experiences (essentially shifting to another state of awareness).

Once you have conducted all the vaporisation you intend to complete for that session, you will find areas of the auric field that seem lacking in sensation or vibrancy—these are shadows, that you will then cleanse. This restores a healthy auric experience, beyond the karmic patterns that were stemming from that point.

Finally, you seal the treatment by restoring the client and yourself back in the treatment environment; transitioning from Karmic State and back into a completed-treatment, conscious state. As you bring together all you have learnt so far into a single treatment method, you will be amazed at the variety and power of these treatments.

Due to the profound nature of Karmic Reiki treatments and the application of The Auric/Karmic Sister symbols, it is advisable to practise treatments several times in a non-professional situation until you are completely confident and comfortable with the technique.

To trigger the Karmic State and conduct a Karmic Reiki treatment, start with your usual connection to the client. After the initial connection, assert internally that this will be a Karmic Reiki treatment and visualise the first symbol, with motion—MKD.

Then begin Reiji Ho and scan the aura for byosen, cold spots or any unusual sensation or synaesthesia. If you find anything, ask yourself "What is this?" If you do not discover an answer straight away, keep asking yourself this same question. It is important to keep asking, regardless of how many times you have already asked. Eventually, the focus you are paying to this question will be rewarded by your subconscious experiences.

Whilst you are asking what have you found in the auric field, continue to examine the form, sensation or synaesthesia, all the time asking the question. As you examine the anomaly, attempt to hone in further information about it—its size, shape, temperature, where it leads, what it is, etc.

Once you have all the information you need, you can either continue to explore further and deciphering new aspects of the object or you can follow the narrative of the karmic pattern/event. Once you are sure you have followed the narrative to a natural conclusion, apply the first symbol (MKD) and vaporise the target until it cannot be felt any more.

Follow this with the second symbol (MTN) to diminish any shadow created from the vaporisation. Finally, use the last symbol (SM) to bring the client back to reality, heat up any karmic chill and smooth the aura.

Whenever you use MKD, be sure to use SM to finish—by using MKD alone, you may finish the treatment with the client feeling quite ill and very cold! You can also use SM by itself if ever the client starts to feel icy cold—this is what's known as a karmic chill. However, this will bring the client out of the Karmic State, effectively ending the treatment.

If you wish to soothe a restless client or if they are in discomfort, opt for MTN as a calming alternative. Only use SM if this does not offer relief. You can always continue a treatment using the traditional methods, Taoist Grace, etc.

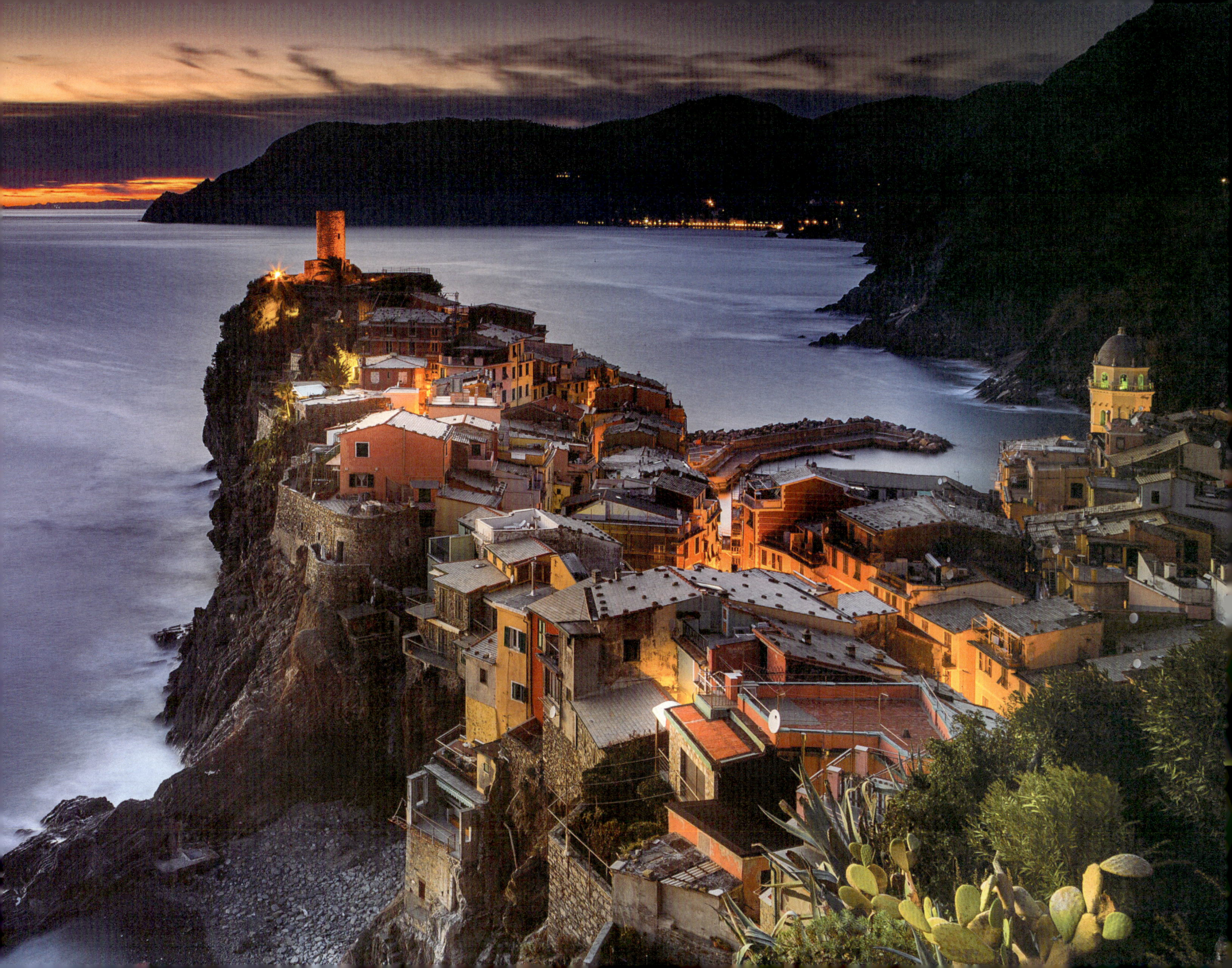

Karmic Vaporiser
MeiKuDo (May Koo Doe)

This powerful perspective works to clear the auric manifestations of physical objects. A rope, knife, water, or brick wall, for example. Its intense nature literally vaporises any connection to that object or event, leaving only a shadow of the karmic pattern.

To apply this perspective, transition by visualising the symbol and the appropriate action (motion) of the symbol—you feel its vibration in your hands or through some other form of synaesthesia. Once you feel this, connect to Reiji Ho and be guided to where you need to work first. When MeiKuDo is complete, use MeiTuNyo to complete the treatment.

Contraindications: It may cause panic attacks as it often creates intense feelings of pressure, fear, or even a sense of dying.

Karmic Shadow Cleanser
MeiTuNyo
(May Too En Joh)

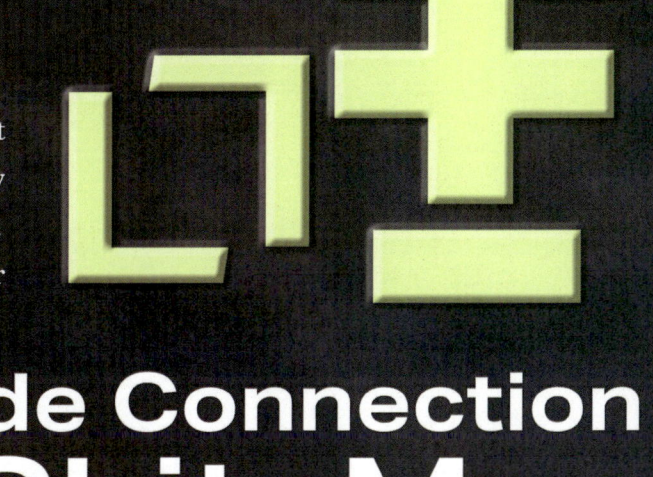

Once a karmic object or event has been detached from the auric experience, it may leave a shadow, or area feeling stagnant/non-existent. To restore a healthy experience here, use MeiTuNyo in the same way as its sister symbol MeiKuDo.

This experience can create bursts of joyous laughter from your client or envelop them with love and feelings of euphoria.

The Guide Connection
ShiteMyo
(She They Me Oh)

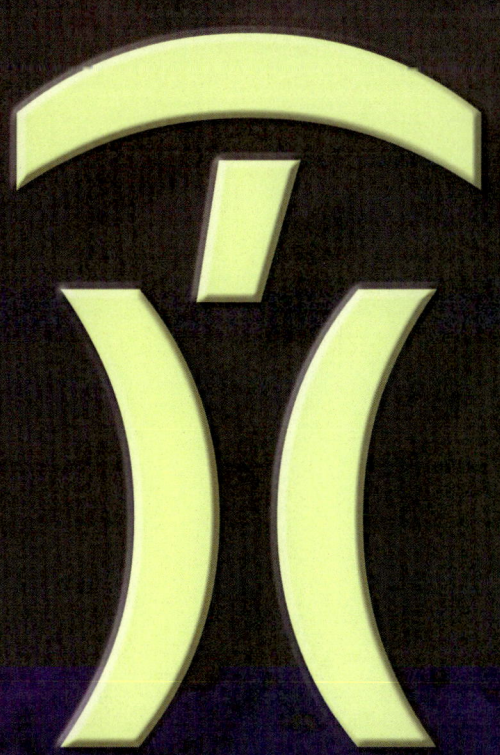

This perspective is, once again, used by the practitioner through visualising the symbol and feeling the results in the hands or through other forms of sensation. It creates a closer connection with the practitioner's subconscious and intuitive ability, as well as forming a deep karmic bond with the client, thus intensifying the treatment.

It works very well in co-dependency (individual and relationships), karmic issues, spiritual growth and anywhere where a formidable sense of compassion and lots of love are needed.

Using this perspective will end a karmic treatment and bring both you and your client back into the physical reality of the environment.

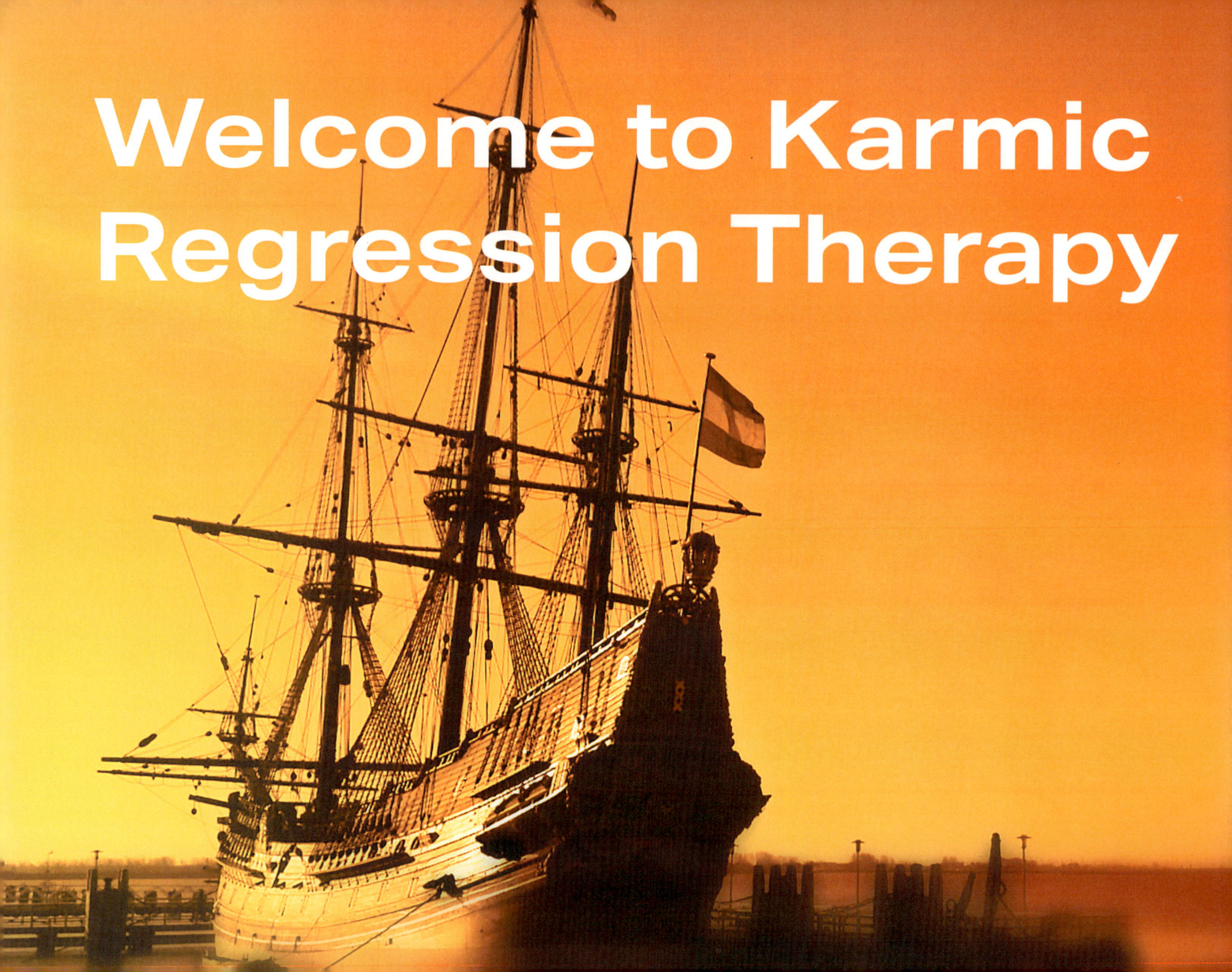

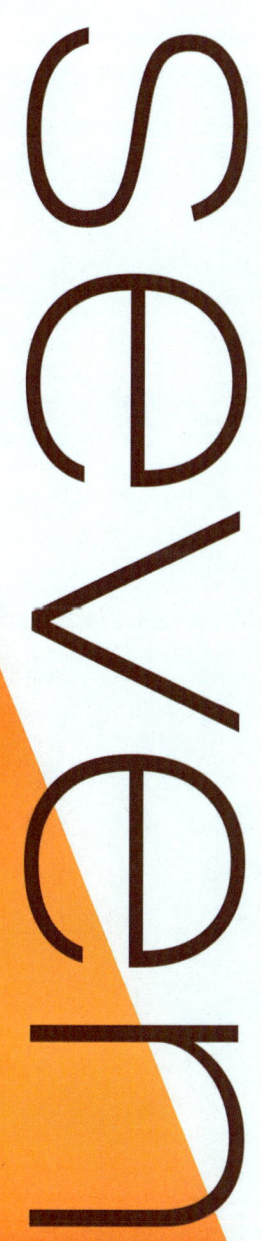

Karmic Reiki, as its name suggests is a form of therapy that is powered by Reiki and focuses on clearing karmic patterns as the means of treatment. The style and technique of treatments, in addition to the powerful experience of Reiki therapy, are very effective when working in this methodology.

However, there are some limitations and drawbacks with Karmic Reiki, and these were addressed in the transition from Karmic Reiki to Karmic Regression Therapy. Overall, these changes affect the driving force behind the therapy, the way treatments are conducted and the philosophy from which treatments are conducted.

The process of entering a Karmic State, clearing and soothing karmic events, etc., and then bringing a client back into the room, remain rather similar to the practice of Karmic Reiki. In KRT treatments, however, we have various philosophies that alter the nature of the events and objects, and the force behind KRT can also feel very different to the experience of Reiki.

One of the biggest differences between Karmic Reiki and KRT appears mainly aesthetic, inasmuch as, similarly to working with Byosen Reikan Ho and Reiji Ho, the practitioner creates a parallel environment or *box* for the treatment to take place within. Thus, instead of walking around the room, using their hands to identify karmic objects, the practitioner sits or stands in one place and uses their hands to work with karma in a contained area.

Having witnessed many years of student practitioners offering Reiki treatments to windows, doors and pot plants, in an attempt to reach the outer extents of a client's auric field, I worked into the methodology a way of treating a person in a micro, mirrored environment.

This introduces an interesting idea because we can understand the box approach as a parallel or mirror of the in-the-room treatment. However, all treatments are parallels or mirrors of what is actually taking place. Whenever you experience hibiki or karmic objects, you are not touching a physical thing. You are entering a gateway into the non-physical universe: what exists beyond our world.

The flow, bounce and vibrations are merely mirrors of some other lifetime, experience or potential reality. Therefore, whether the box is between your hands or in the room, it is still—and always will be—a box! Even when you are using hand positions with a client, or on yourself with self-treatment, it is still a box; one that mirrors another place in time, or beyond time.

Defining a set environment for your treatments to take place within is so much better for various reasons. Firstly, the logistical processes of treatment—holding your hand above your head to Reiki the top of a bookcase is more tiring than holding your hands out in front of you.

Walking round the room several times is more tiring for you and more distracting for your client than sitting or standing in one place. Focusing your treatment in one small, defined area is more effective than prancing around the room, *waving your arms in the air like you just don't care.* This is a professional treatment, not the Macarena!

All joking aside, when we look deeper at the processes of KRT, we realise that the evolution from Karmic Reiki is far more than simply the appearance of treatment styles. The box environment creates a powerful arena that is smaller in dimensions than you are. When you work with issues that are bigger than you, they seem bigger than you—treat issues as small, they become small and easier to treat!

It is important to remember that by making things smaller we may lose the nuance or detail within the treatment environment—this is where an ever-increasing sensitive and commitment to improving your senses is vital to KRT Box Treatments.

Then, we have the methodology improvements—extrapolating, refining, and adapting the Three Sisters into a six-step Karmic Regression Therapy system is far more robust. Each step is about honing in on a specific aspect of treatment and targeting that experience. In all energy therapies, the big picture is easy, it is the detail that is often lacking.

However, just as a game of *Jenga* involves the tower falling when you remove a single brick; KRT can reduce karmic trauma to dust when you target the precise event that causes the trauma in the first place. The practitioner tools of KRT were designed with this in mind.

When we look to the difference in treatment, you may wonder what you need to learn or do differently to master the KRT

Box treatment method. The wondrous thing is Box Treatments are actually easier and expend less effort for greater results.

The challenge is that your sensory and intuitive abilities need to be honed to work within the box. Whereas feeling an object and watching your hands define it in the air is fairly easy when you get the hang of it, using your synaesthesia and mind-abilities to interpret the treatment feedback takes practice.

There is real mastery in the practitioner who can move beyond what their hands are doing to work purely emotionally and cerebrally. However, once you do master that ability, it is very powerful and will come as naturally to you as recalling your own name.

The more practised, sensitive, and intuitive you are with Byosen Reikan Ho and Reiji Ho, the easier KRT Box Treatments will be to grasp. And, if you are experiencing real challenges with the box, focus on these two traditional aspects of our therapy rather than trying to force the box method. Practising your sensitivity of hibiki and the free-flow of Reiji Ho will hone your skills in readiness for effective Box Treatments.

With this in mind, let us work at creating a Box environment. The first step is to calibrate to the first KRT orientation. This will enable you to trigger the following perspectives of KRT and define your Arena for treatment.

KRT—The Practitioner Tools

The Arena
Trigger name: Arena, said three times.

The Arena defines your neutral space—the location of your treatment in space and time. this is usually visualised in the shape of a box and placed on your lap, although you could alter the shape according to your personal preference—spheres, pyramids or more complex shapes are all equally purposeful.

This aspect of the box creation develops an arena for treatment—one that highlights karmic events and distinguishes these from the physical environment. The more you come to know your own experiences within the Arena, the better you will discern karmic patterns, events and objects.

The Arena remains neutral throughout the treatment, as you mirror the patterns of your client's auric field across it. The Arena is like a blank canvas that never interferes with the other vibrations that are contained within, yet counteracts any *external* interference.

The Primer
Trigger Name: Prime, said three times.

This KRT tool shifts our perspective of the auric field to prime us for treatment. By creating this layer of treatment, we increase our sensitivity to environmental vibrations, especially those of the aura, and fine-tune our synaesthesia abilities to interpret what those vibrations are hinting at.

The Primer also helps your intuitive abilities when treating, specifically in the range of karmic (miasmatic, holographic and Viridian) work. This eases the intuitive translation of vibrations into tangible experiences that you can then relate to your client in feedback sessions.

The Sensing

Trigger Name: Sense, said three times.

The Sensing perspective is the main tool of KRT, one that will help you to sense what is happening in your primed Arena. The effect of this tool is rather like turning up the volume on your sensory experience. In one way, this increase in force will mean you can identify experiences with greater ease, however the way in which the tool works will also help you to sense the more nuanced details of the treatment.

To understand this better, the increase in power occurs with the weaker or hidden aspects of the treatment, while the already powerful vibrations remain at their existing level. Overall, therefore, we experience a balancing in the experience that helps us to sense more and at deeper layers of karma, miasma, etc.

The Clearing

Trigger Name: Cleanse, said three times.

Once you have located a karmic object, or event in the arena, you can decipher this and then clear it, using the clearing tool to literally vaporise or diminish the vibrations involved. This tool removes force from the vibration, meaning that it can be disconnected from, with the minimum of stress or reaction.

At the Viridian degree of treatment, we come to appreciate what happens to vibrations that exit without force. For now, however, it is useful to know these vaporised vibrations cease to exist in the physical universe in any conscious or sensory way.

The Soothing
Trigger Name: Soothe, said three times.

Once karmic patterns have been negated, you can activate the soothing tool to ensure that everything is smoothed over. The experiences that now relate to your client's life are now much more conducive to their happiness and success, whilst the disconnection from karmic events, miasma, etc., continue to occur at a deeper level.

The healing process can be challenging, with the KRT treatment usually triggering a detoxification process, the soothing will ensure this period of cleansing happens quickly, effectively and as pleasantly as possible.

The Sealing
Trigger Name: Seal, said three times.

The Sealing tool is used to seal the treatment into place. Whenever we treat a client with any form of energy therapy, the more focused and defined the treatment, the more powerful the results will be. By sealing the treatment, you are effectively stating that only the experiences contained within that particular treatment box form a part of the healing process.

This can seem limiting at first, but remember the *Jenga* brick analogy and you will see how only targeting that brick is more effective than a diluted, catch-all treatment that is expected to work on everything... regardless of whether it has been defined or not!

This tool ensures that all the work done within the treatment Box is maintained for as long as possible and that all smoothing and soothing is held in place, whilst any detoxification occurs during the twenty-one days post-treatment.

This three-week period after treatment is an important time when monitoring how effective the treatment has been, appreciating how a treatment has evolved or changed your client's auric experiences.

A three-week time period is rather specific and is due to the chemical nature of the detoxification that takes place after a treatment. When the vibrational work translates to physical changes, via the natural processes of the body, our balance of neurochemicals changes. This routine is very natural and is part of the healing process—once complete, your client will feel much better than prior to the treatment.

This detoxification process only affects a small number of people, and only some of the time. In the majority of cases, you will feel great after the treatment. The process is also called an Energy Alignment Process, or EAP.

The Foundation Treatment Method

This basic method for creating a treatment box (also known as an Arena Environment), is to define your box, between your hands, using each tool in turn to create the arena, prime the experience, sense the specific events for treatment, vaporise the events, soothe the experience, and seal the Arena.

When treating, you will experience sensations of flowing, swirling, bouncy, electrical or magnetic forces. These may be subtle and intangible or very real, almost physical in nature and form. The more you practise feeling the sensations of flow and bounce, the more detail you will be able to translate.

The better the translation from vibration to synaesthesia, the more feedback you can offer your client and the greater depth of experience you will share. By the time you take on your first clients, you will need to sense both flow and bounce, interpret and experience Karmic State and be able to communicate your discoveries in a professional and supportive way to your clients.

Technique:

- Start by standing (or sitting), with your hands on either side of your client's head around the temple area, creating a connection with your client.
- If you wish to do so, ask for higher guidance of some kind to support you during this treatment.
- Now continue by triggering the *Primer* tool.
- After a few minutes, you should begin to feel a really good connection with your partner. You can then trigger the *Sensing* tool and start to move the experience of their auric field through the box, using your hands to decipher the flows/bounce.
- As you locate different dynamics, distortions and disruptions, constantly ask yourself "What is this?", "How did it get here?", "Where is it from?" and so on. Be aware of any synaesthetic response you attain and use these responses as a *way into* the karmic experience (story).
- Once you have exhausted the experience of an object, use the *Clearing* until the object is diminished.
- After that, work for a further two-to-three minutes with the *Soothing* and *Sealing* before venturing on to the next object.
- Once you have completed the main elements of the treatment, work with the *Sealing* for another five minutes or so.
- Finally, bring your partner fully back into the room.

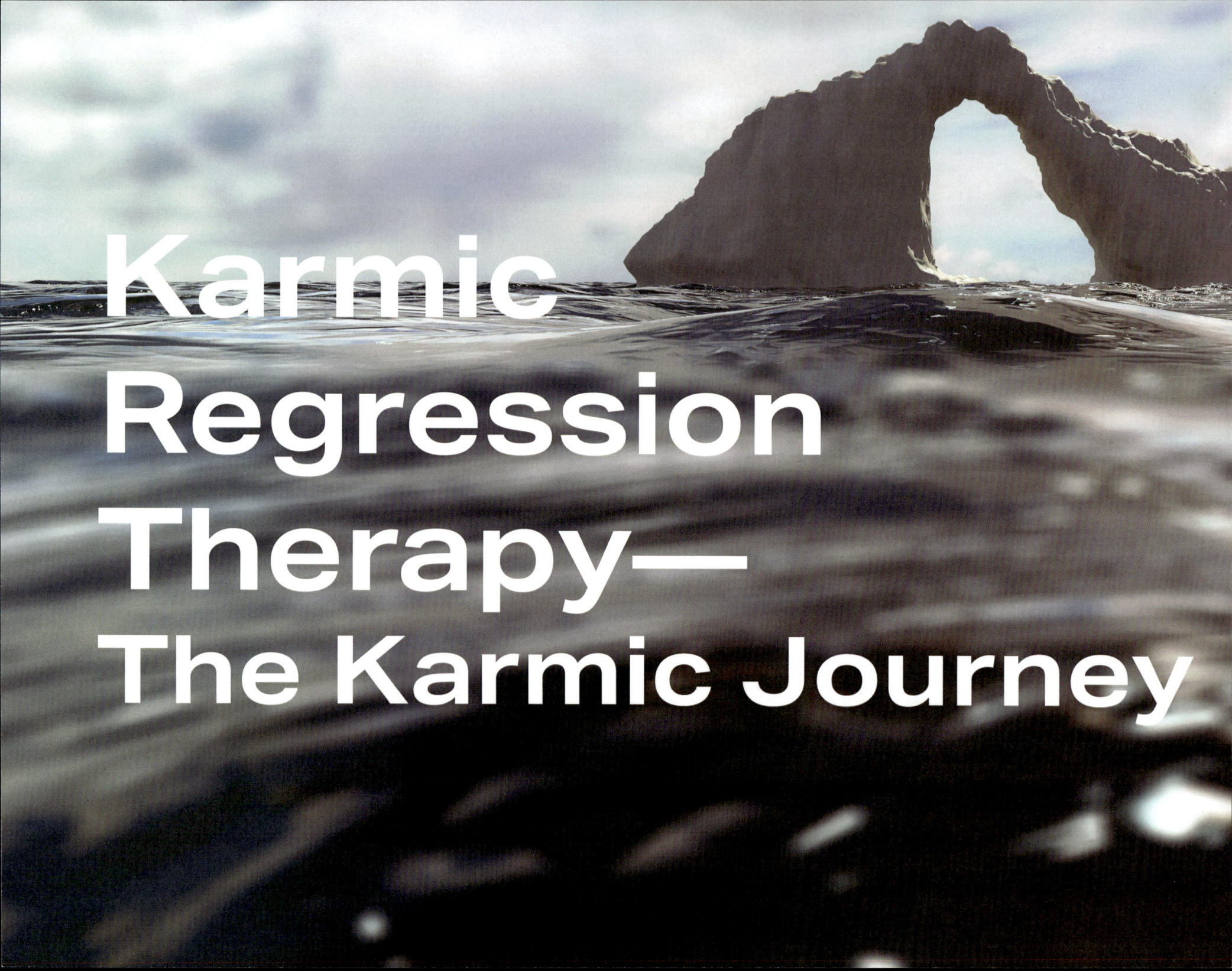

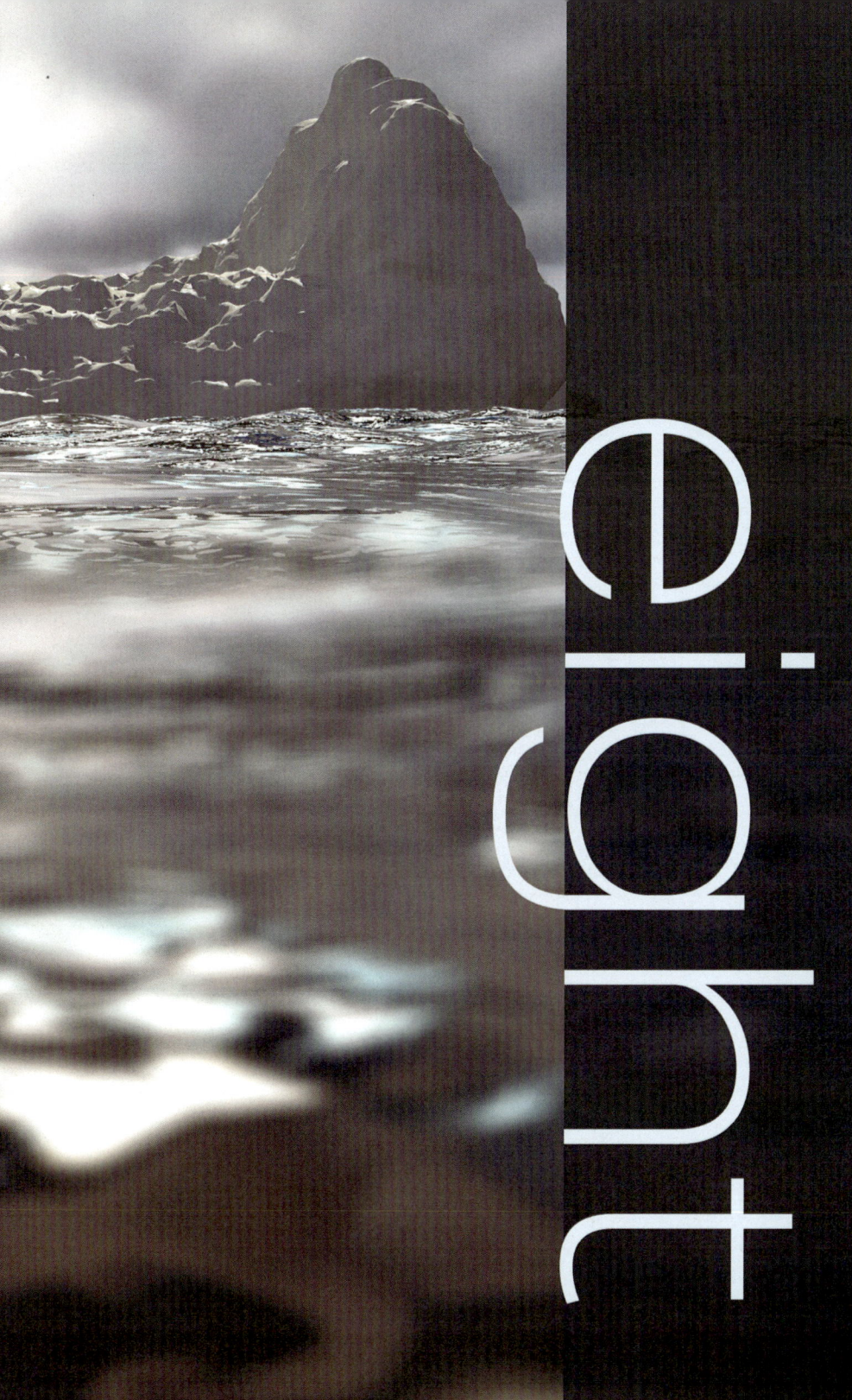

eight

Throughout your practitioner experience, your foundation Box Treatment method will be at the core of your professional experiences. However, the ethos that drives your Box Treatments will differ greatly from degree to degree, starting with a karmic perspective and working towards a Viridian perspective.

At each degree, we adapt the treatment to embrace the terminology and concepts of that specific degree, whilst retaining a universal treatment style. From a training perspective, this makes your learning journey one of practising and practising the Box Treatment method until you are confident to make the small philosophical adjustments to your therapeutic practice.

Starting with the concept of karma, we are looking to identify the common themes between the different degrees and use them as a framework that adapts as you move from one degree to the other. For instance, the concept of a single soul going on a journey through many incarnations may, on the face of it, seem very different from ancestral miasma.

Here, vibrations of trauma and dis-ease are transferred from parent to child, becoming more and more diluted with each generation. This dilution process alters the vibrations, making their underlying effects stronger and more profound with each lifetime.

Many new students of KRT resist this ethos with extreme fervour because they are fixated on both viewpoints' dogmas and miss the integral, core messages they share: those of a soul, vibration, energy, force, experiences, consciousness, through many lifetimes.

Beyond this core ethos, our own internal imagery takes over and depicts either a neatly packaged soul or a long stream of flowing vibrations. One bounces along from body to body, while the other flows through bodies and lifetimes. In foundation terms, however, energy does not bounce or flow. It exists as a Universal Constant that simply changes form in space and time, depending on the reality.

This backbone principle of energy and the experience of life moulds the true heart of KRT. In the first two degrees, we see lifetimes in a more linear fashion; in the last two, the lifetimes become potential or possible life experiences. Either way, we come back to energy and life; within the perspective of time and beyond time.

To explore a deeper layer of KRT and the underlying principles of karma, we will partake in a whirlwind adventure through the traditional Buddhist view of karma and the karmic cycle. Whilst this is a greatly simplified view of the complex processes depicted in Buddhist philosophy, we are looking to create a foundation of practice, and not a comprehensive perspective of the spiritual principles involved.

The Twelve Links of Dependent Origination depict the soul's journey across millennia, which in turn develops the wider context— the lifetime of your body serving as a culture for the soul as it travels through many bodies, many lifetimes.

These twelve stages of the evolution through a single lifetime begin with ignorance and end in death. Each of the intervening stages sculpts the person's lifetime and its effects on the broader context. The Twelve Links of Dependent Origination are:

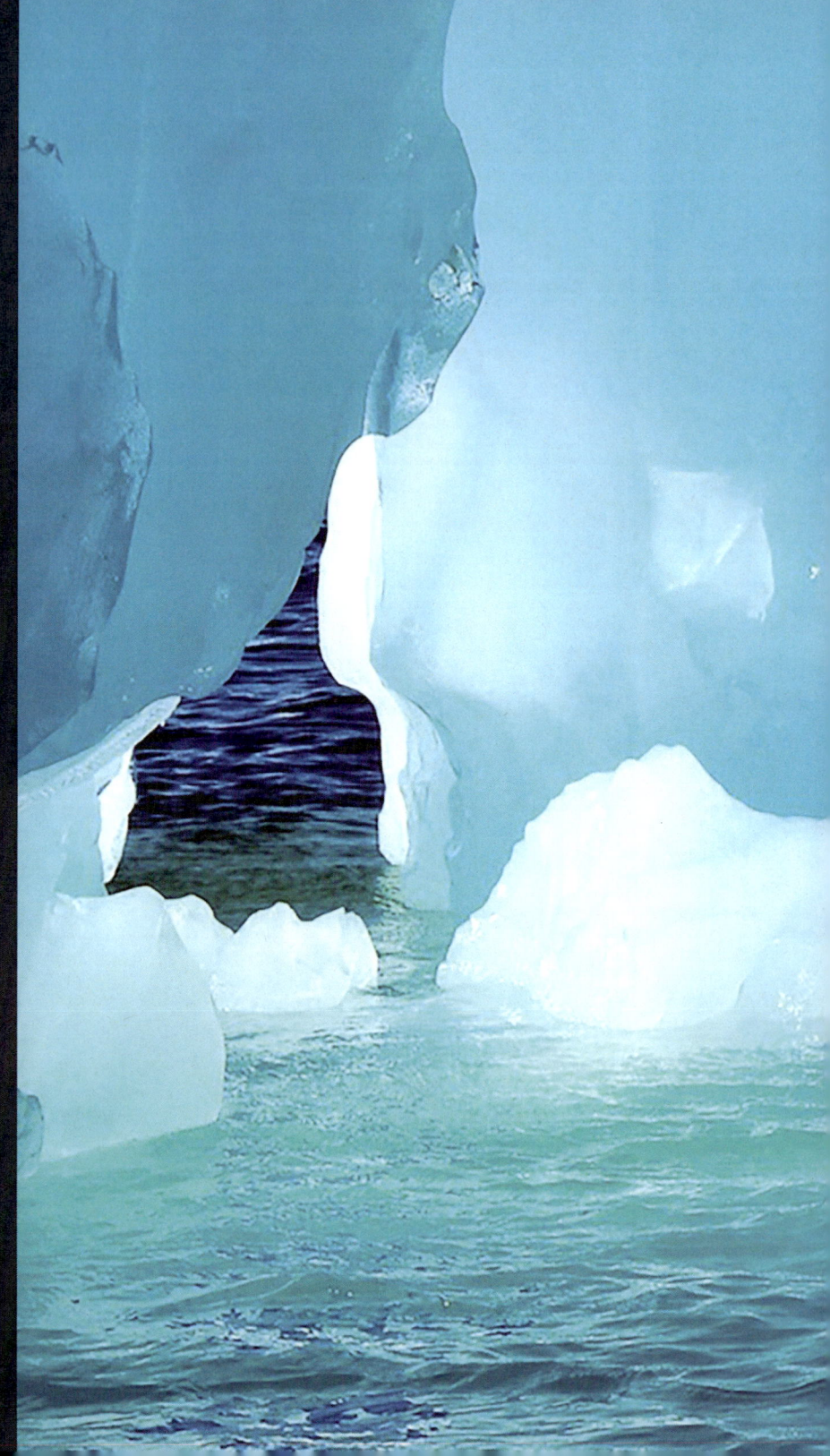

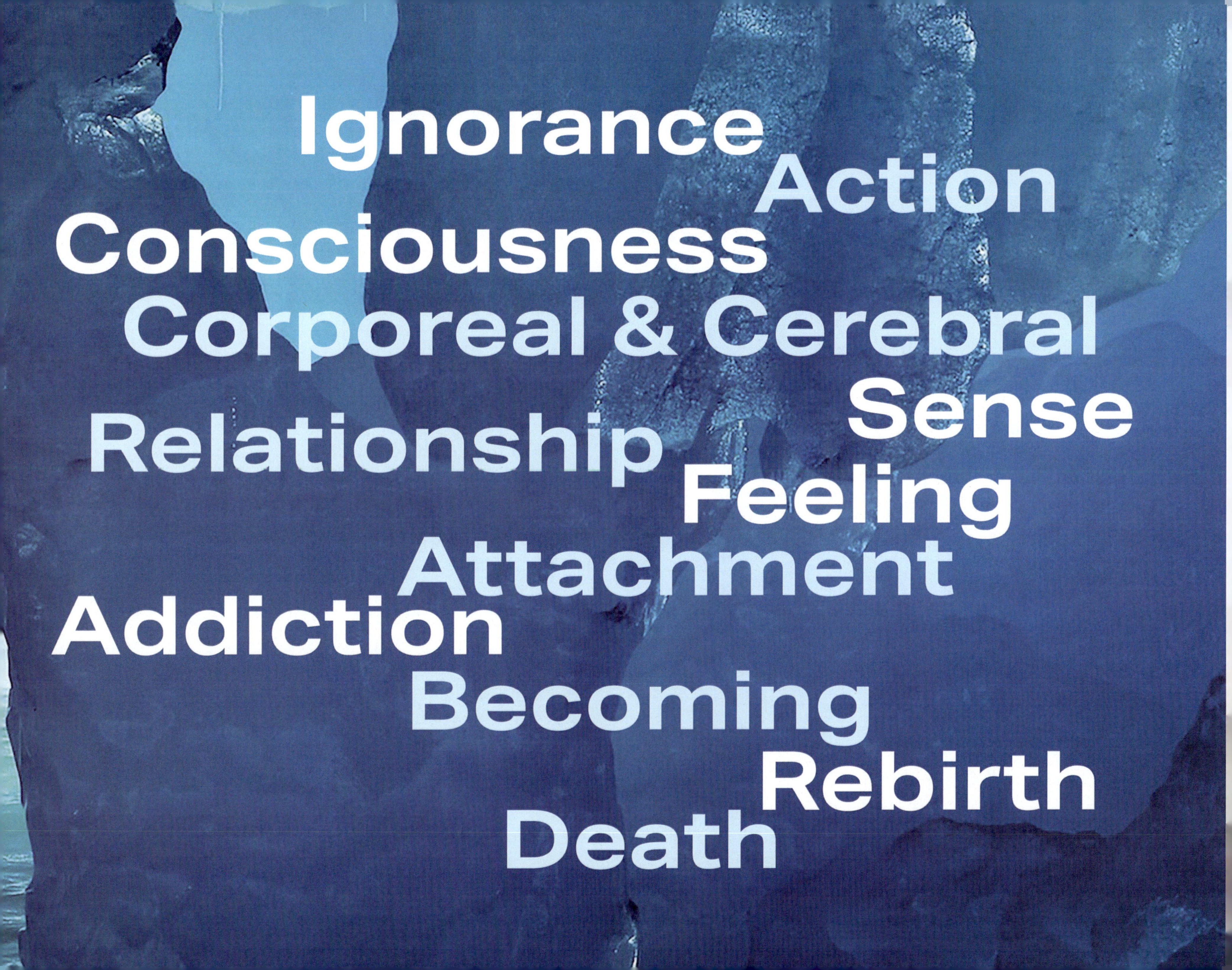

Ignorance

Action

Consciousness

Corporeal & Cerebral

Sense

Relationship

Feeling

Attachment

Addiction

Becoming

Rebirth

Death

Beginning with **ignorance**, we exist without knowledge, and this lack of wisdom is the cause of all pain and trauma. We do not know ourselves and our own potential; we are blind to the true nature of the soul and how we are a force of pure will.

Transcending our own ignorance requires **action**, and it is in this action that we cause the effects of karma. The actions of the past create the present karma we are currently experiencing, and the acts of the present create future karma. Action could be a thought, a spoken word or an actual deed.

Consciousness refers to the Eight Degrees of Consciousness (six in some traditions.) These different layers of conscious experience encompass a traditional view of the five senses (sight, hearing, touch, taste, and smell), the subconscious, waking consciousness and deep karma or superconsciousness.

The **corporeal and cerebral** experience underpins our psychological and physical existence; from the experience of form, feelings, perceptions, and mental imagery to our conscious awareness of these. The Five Aggregates weave together the corporeal world and our cerebral understanding of that world.

The **senses** or *six bases* are simply the eye, ear, nose, tongue, touch, and cerebral function. These are the physical tools that present us with feedback about the world and our positioning within it.

The **relationship** between our consciousness and another physical form within the contextual experience of time, is the very thing that enables us to appreciate a separateness within the world and our place amongst everything around us. It is in this relationship we distinguish a thing as pleasurable, painful or neutral.

As we sense and experience the different objects and elements of the physical world, we form **feelings** towards those things. In some cases these feelings may be pleasurable or painful, whilst other things cause no feeling one way or the other (a neutral reaction). Upon these feelings, we develop a strong desire towards pleasurable things and an avoidance desire away from pain.

Attachment is a psychological state that increases the experience of our desires, forming habitual patterns around certain objects or elements of life. This mental longing for a thing creates an intense need that exists without ever attaining satisfaction.

The attachments we form create **addiction**, which consists of four stronger, more compulsive forms of desire. These are: desired objects, view of the self, morality and behaviour, and damaging perspectives. These addictions are always detrimental, causing the effect of traumatic future karma.

Becoming fully-realised in life, through the development of an actualised karma brings us to a new phase of the journey. When we accept the full-potential of ourselves and our karma, we enter into a blissful, deeply spiritual stage of this lifetime.

The **rebirth** is sometimes understood in connection to the act of having children or becoming a parent. However, it can also pertain to a metaphorical rebirth such as a spiritual awakening, the creation of a legacy or the complete and irrevocable change of one's life. Once the rebirth phase is complete, we begin to decay.

The final link of a single lifetime is **death**. It is not really an aspect of life but something that occurs after life is complete. As we enter into the death phase the cycle begins again, and the effect of our karma determines the course of the soul's next lifetime.

Another fundamental aspect of karma is the Six Realms of Desire, which relate to the conditioned existence of *Samsara*. Samsara is brought about through karma or action. In other words, these allegories describe the nature of one's existence, as determined by karma, and they are tenuously related to the ideas of heaven and hell found in various religious belief systems.

The first realm is that of the Deva or gods. Here, beings of immense power live, grow old and die having led lives of colossal status. They are so omnipotent they are blind to the suffering of others and, despite their long lives, demonstrate neither wisdom nor compassion for anyone. When they die, Devas are reincarnated into one of the other realms.

The realm of the Titans is home to a different type of powerful being, presented as enemies of the Devas. Driven by jealousy and rage, the Titans look down upon others, being blinded by envy. Living a life of hatred and jealousy will lead to reincarnation in this realm, destined to want, but never to have.

Next is the realm of Hungry Ghosts, where these beings starve in torment. These unfortunate creatures crave nourishment and pleasure but never receive either—mainly because they are looking outside of themselves to replenish their hunger. Those who live an addicted life or are driven by compulsion/obsession often find themselves reincarnated here.

The Hell realm is the most terrifying and worst of all. The inhabitants of hell are aggressive and angry; they inflicted their rage on others through extreme displays of horrible temper. As a consequence, they end up isolated and unable to accept kindness or love. Those who spend their lives angry and aggressive towards others are reborn into hell.

The realm of Animals is said to house those governed by stupidity, prejudice, and complacency—those who live a life ruled by base instincts, having never tried to get past the ignorance into which we all are born. Those who live a sheltered life, blinded by stupid ideals and their own dogma are reincarnated into this realm.

Finally, we visit the human realm, where beings may escape Samsara and reach a state of enlightenment. Only a few ever reach for that Moksha (liberation from Samsara) and recognise their own ability to achieve it. As the only realm that enables us to attain enlightenment, this realm is seen as a real gift for the souls that pass through. To reincarnate here, you must demonstrate a life of passion, desire or doubt.

Whilst many interpret these realms as real places, we could view the realms as layers of human existence. Here, in our physical world, those who live their lives envying others exist in the realm of Titans, whilst those who are always hungry for more are Hungry Ghosts. It is only through living a life of passion, doubt, or desire that we enter the Human realm and have the opportunity to strive for enlightenment.

In the Human realm, we see four distinct layers of behaviour; those who seek to learn about their path and the way forward; those who reach enlightenment by themselves; those who are destined for enlightenment through their self-belief and by knowing their own nature; and those who have seen into their future and have forgotten the ego-self.

With these layers in mind we begin to realise that anybody who is not in the path of these layers exists within the Human realm outside of these layers or in one of the other realms.

One very important consideration is that we need to be keenly aware of ourselves and how we present the concept of karma to others. The traditions from which karma stems are ancient; they have existed for thousands of years. However, in our modern society, it is easy to misinterpret the karmic journey, especially when speaking to a person who exists outside the Human realm.

Furthermore, telling an abuse survivor their experiences stem from bad karma or commenting to relatives who have just lost a loved one that the death they mourn was a result of their karmic actions is not only unprofessional, it is extremely inappropriate on just about every possible level! Reconciling karma with an ongoing situation is a very challenging endeavour and will often result in blame.

Think for a moment how easy it is to blame other people, to blame the, past and even to blame oneself. Making the shift from blame to responsibility is a far more productive perspective. More importantly, when you gather your own areas of responsibility around you, you can determine what you can change and what you cannot change.

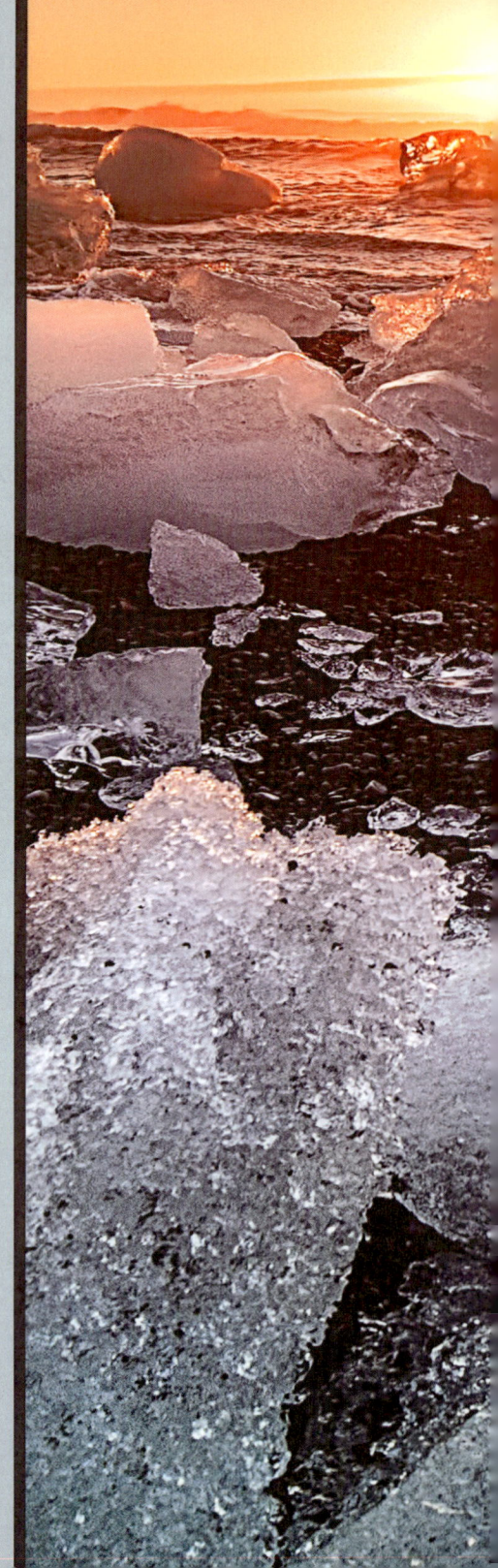

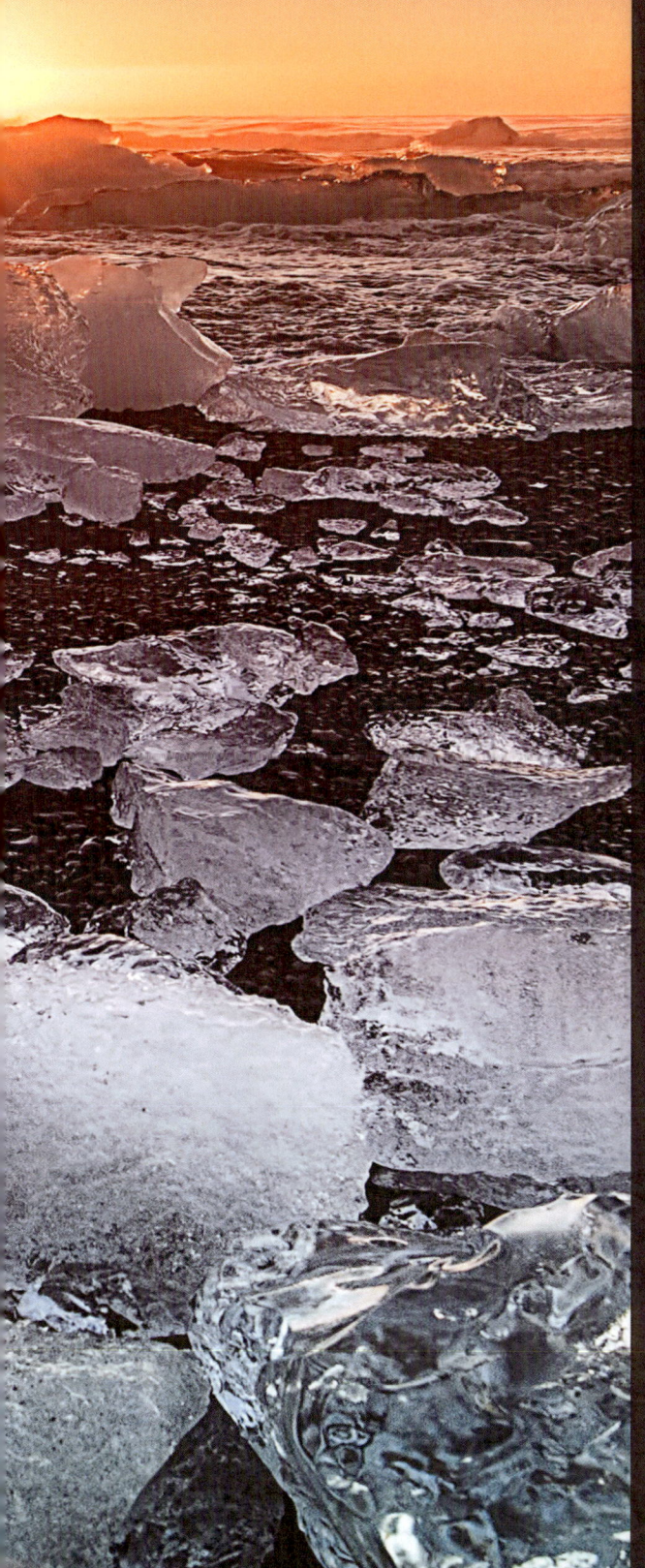

For any person, blaming their parents for events that occurred in childhood often comes naturally and, indeed, the parents are responsible for those events. However, when a person is 40-years-old and is still blaming their parents for the choices and behaviour they themselves are making, it is time for some self-accountability.

As children, we are taught one set of perspectives of life from our parents but, as adults, we are responsible for looking at our lives and deciding whether that set of perspectives is appropriate or if we need to shift to a new set of perspectives.

Expanding on this idea, when we blame karma for events in the present, we are removing our own accountability for what we could do differently and blame something we can do nothing about. This idea provides us with a very important foundation for KRT treatments conducted in space and time.

When we clear karmic events (and the like), we are acting in the present and taking responsibility for our present. This action does not rewrite or change the past, for we are not accountable for that past. This leads us to a startling shift of perspective when we apply the same method to karmic patterns and the traditional allegories of the karmic journey.

When we understand that karma is of the present moment, not of the past, we realise that we are not to blame; nobody is to blame. However, we are all accountable for our own actions in the present moment.

A karmic pattern, rather than being a habit that exists through time, is one we are connected to in that specific moment—which then becomes one connected to all points in time. That expression of hatred is not a karmic pattern from two hundred years ago—it is a current connection to the Titan realm that floods our experience with hatred (and flows out through time to create hatred through time).

It is important to remember the realms are metaphorical, even though when you are connected to the Hell realm, you feel as if you are in hell; and, when connected to the Deva realm you feel on top of the world and may even feel better than other people! Our experiences, over time, have become enveloped by the imagery, story, and metaphor of the karmic journey.

Appreciating how our actions at the moment are reflected throughout time is the very first step in understanding the Viridian perspective of life beyond time. Where traditions see a chain of events that exist within the context of time, the KRT practitioner views karma as a momentary, fleeting thing that is all-encompassing when connected to a particular aspect of the journey.

When acting from the realm of Hungry Ghosts, a person will contort their life around a certain craving. When they are stuck in the Animal realm, they will seem ignorant and their views will make your jaw drop at how ridiculously blind a person could be. When a person is passing through the Human realm, they will be driven by passion and desire, yet riddled with doubt—however, at this point they can transcend Samsara into enlightenment.

Remember, even though we use the term *Human realm*, it refers to a metaphor, not a reality—all people are humans, regardless of which realm they are currently acting from. And, as therapists, we strive to act within the Human realm, but are also just as likely to function from any other realm—and, if you believe you are invulnerable to karma, you are probably situated at this moment in the Deva realm!

How does this translate to the treatment of karmic patterns in KRT? Well, in the Karmic Reiki perspective we are looking to treat the current connections to karmic events from the past (those past events, from past lives, that are currently affecting us at this moment). In KRT, we shift to a perspective of being completely in the present—if a person is experiencing a link to a karmic pattern, this is not a past life event, but a contemporary perspective of one of the Karmic realms.

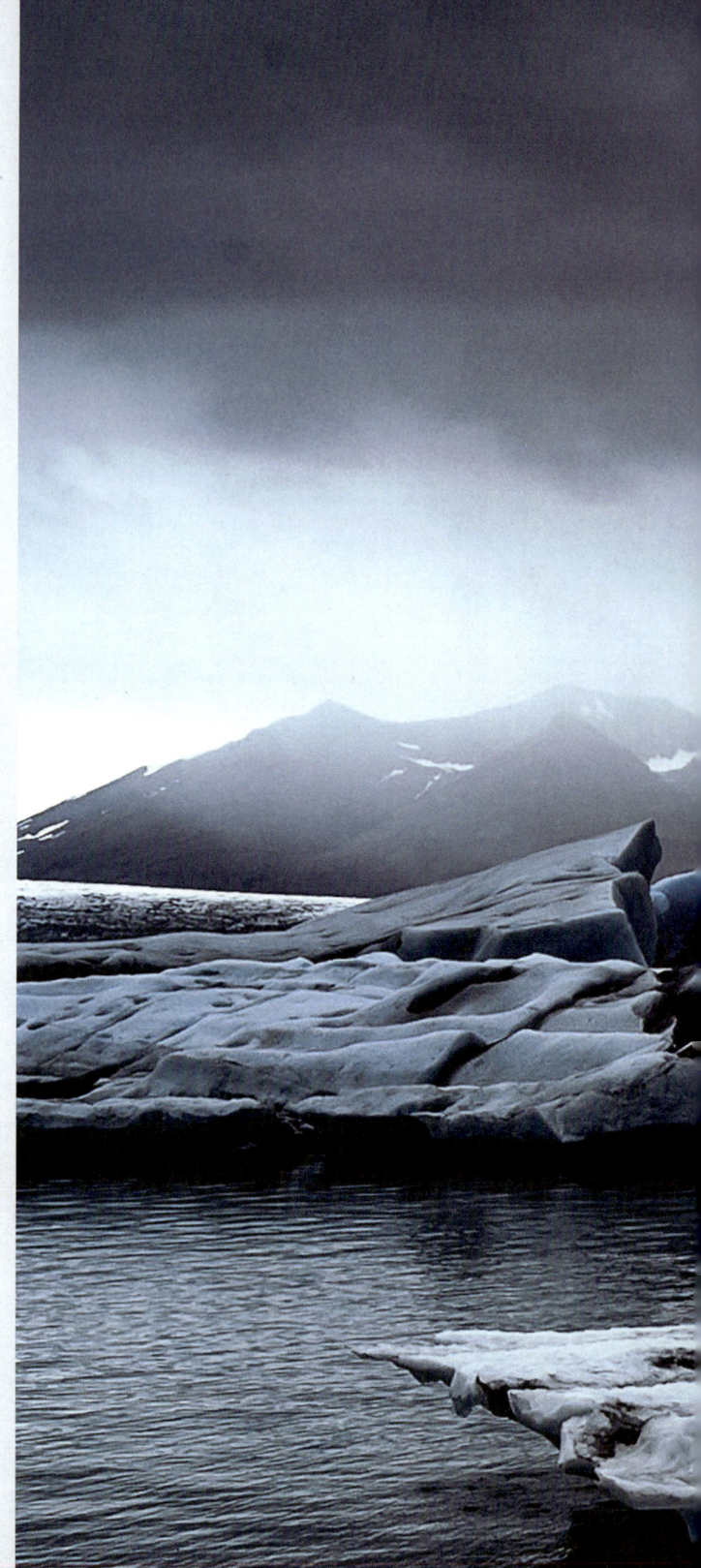

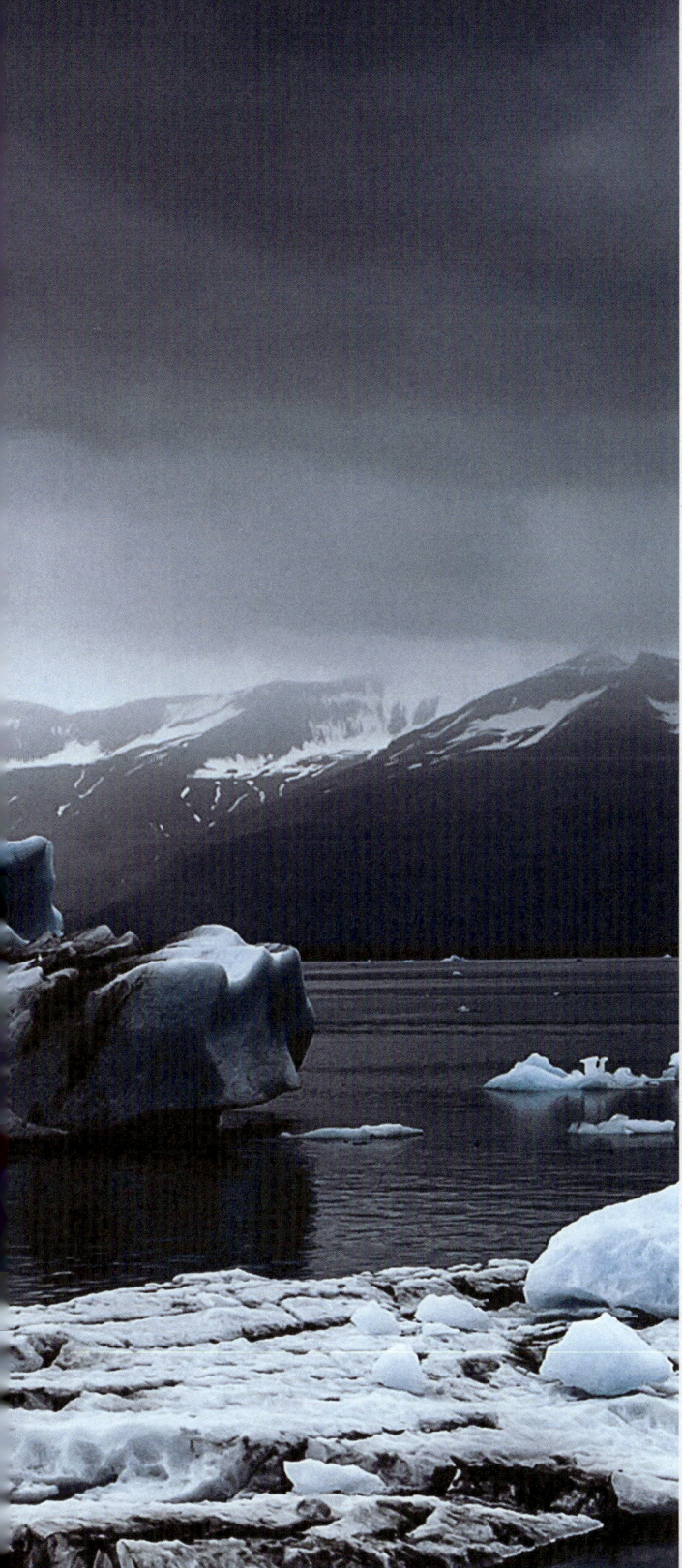

We seek to clear the objects, events and other karmic experiences to shift the client into the Human realm. We then seek to equip them with a way forward; towards the release of Samsara and the acceptance of enlightenment.

We can still talk in terms of past lives. However, do keep in mind that the entire concept of a past life enables the client to relinquish their accountability in the present, whilst blaming the past for all their troubles. Regressing a person through the Links of Dependent Origination is a far more effective way of appreciating the way KRT successfully clears karmic patterns.

A client's actions may be connecting them to the Titan realm, but their consciousness has not yet realised this. As a consequence, they cannot differentiate between themselves, their actions, and the karmic pattern. Their senses cannot define it, and their comprehension of the relationship they are having with the Titan realm will not be apparent enough for them to move beyond it.

When a client is attached or even addicted to their place within a realm—they cannot bear to be around people (Hell), crave cigarettes (Hungry Ghosts), or compulsively express sexist, racist or homophobic attitudes (Animal)—they need to transition beyond these karmic patterns to fully enter the becoming and rebirth phases. KRT can help you support them in this endeavour.

In summary, when conducting your foundation treatments, seek to identify the events, objects and patterns that are currently presenting themselves through the Box Arena, and understand these in terms of which realm they stem from and how your client is relating to them (Links of Dependent Origination).

This will enable you to offer very sophisticated feedback that will truly inspire your client to heal. This also means that, once cleared, the karmic pattern is less likely to return, as it supported by the feedback you have offered and the awareness of the karmic challenges you have highlighted for your client.

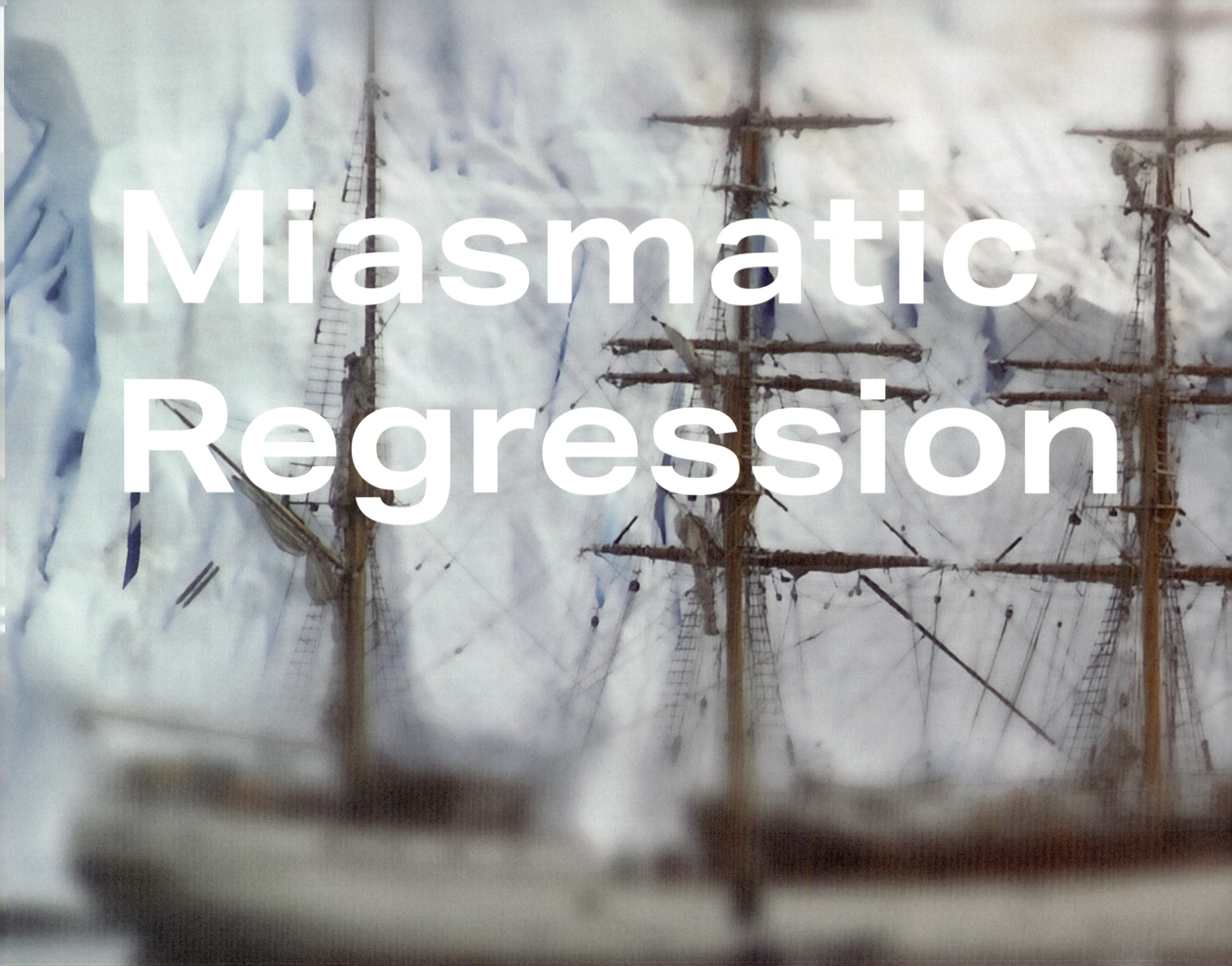

The **miasma** of Victorian London was **accredited** with a whole slew of dis-eases from **typhoid** to cholera.

nine

The Victorians believed that clouds of bad air flowed through the streets of The Old Smoke. Should one breathe in these miasmatic fumes, they would be struck down with some terrible affliction.

The real problem was down to unhygienic streets and the complete lack of effective sewage treatment—a situation that was rectified by an enormous project to construct London's underground sewerage system. Yet, the idea of a miasma or *miasm* remained in terms of vibrational therapy.

Instead of polluting the air, the vibrational miasma is a fog around the person's wellbeing; permeating their natural state of health through vibrations that flow from generation to generation. Common forms of miasm include skin dis-eases such as leprosy, sexual health dis-eases, syphilis, and gonorrhoea, and respiratory dis-eases such as TB. In modern terms, new miasms have developed, such as radiation/petrochemical, vaccination and HIV/AIDS.

The development of a dis-ease in one individual means they pass on the vibration or miasm of that dis-ease to their offspring. Each time the miasm is passed on, the vibration is diluted—which somewhat counterintuitively makes the miasm stronger. A centuries-old miasm will have an increasingly powerful hold over each generation until cleared.

In various forms of vibrational medicine including KRT, we can decipher the miasmatic causes of a person's current issues. By identifying their symptoms, we can trace a root cause to a specific miasm. There are four main miasms (or miasmas, or miasmatas) in KRT and several secondary miasms that were defined later as a way of encompassing developments in society, culture and how dis-eases have changed over time.

The four main miasmatic forms are:

Psoric Sycotic Syphilitic Tubercular

The secondary forms are:

Cancer Acute Thyroid Ringworm Malaria Leprosy HIV/AIDS Petrochemical

The **Psoric** miasm generally manifests itself through the dis-ease of one's body to external and environmental factors. Stimuli such as light, noise, and aromas create imbalances and dysfunction in the individual. These are often indicative of themes such as headaches, nausea and discomfort.

A person affected by this miasm will usually struggle to succeed. They will suffer from anxiety and doubt their ability to achieve, but will also hope for success. They see failure as a step on the path and will pick themselves up after a major setback. However, they frequently struggle to support themselves.

The Psoric personality traits can manifest as optimism. The person will make the effort and get the job done, although the opposite may also be true, inasmuch as they may give up easily, drowning in despair and a deep lack of self-confidence. They will struggle with the world and experience extreme highs and lows. Fearful, insecure and constantly anxious, they will be exceptionally alert and stressed.

There is often a toxic relationship with money and a struggle for wealth, because of poverty. They may become greedy and materialistic in striving for well-being and success. Their immune system is frequently compromised, and they

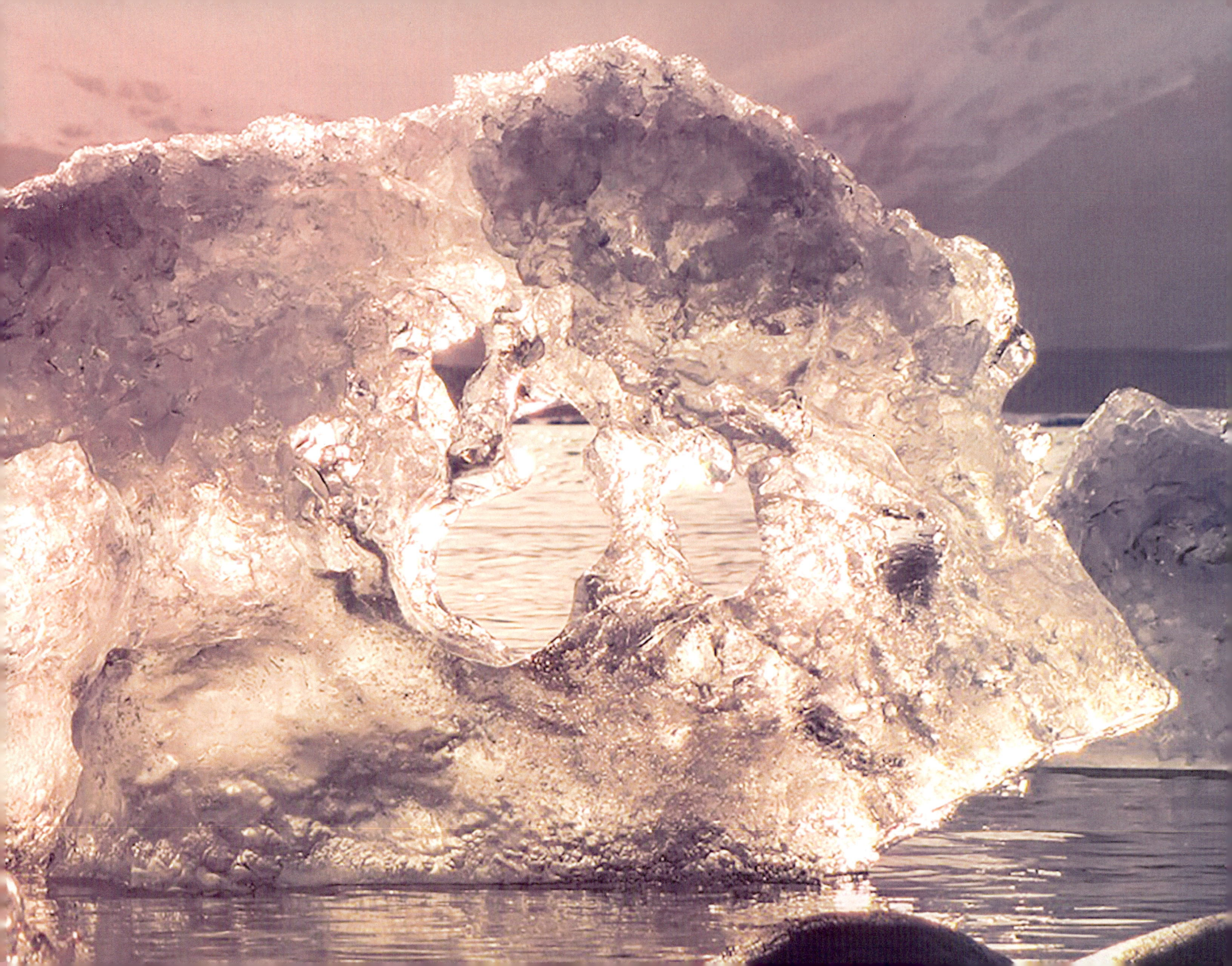

will have frequent colds, flu, injuries, etc. Change is also important here, as life changes will often cause dis-ease or the effects of the miasm to be aggravated.

The **Sycotic** miasm (not to be confused with psychotic), usually manifests as sensitivity to specific issues such as weakness, lack or limitations. As they attempt to transcend these factors, they will encounter symptoms such as tumours, allergies, warts, asthma, and skin issues.

The person's tendency to overcompensate will become apparent through fixed and fixated behaviour. Rigid ideas and obsessive, ritualistic behaviour leads to hypersensitive reactions to many things and a very restricted lifestyle. They will often become lost in guilt, remorse, self-reproach and a fear of being exposed.

There is a connection between this miasm and the suppression of gonorrhoea at some point in their heritage. They will often weep when spoken to, anticipating words that cause them anxiety or upset. They are secretive and hide things from others; suspicious, jealous and forgetful, this person is difficult to trust or rely upon.

Their obsessive habits usually present themselves with overly-frequent hand washing and other features of OCD behaviour. They may be timid in nature, avoid issues that challenge them, and will submit to the slightest confrontation.

The **Syphilitic** miasm is destructive, unmanageable and seemingly hopeless. The symptoms are drastic and devastating. Tissue degeneration, gangrene, and ulceration are just some ways this miasm manifests in the person. They will usually descend into a complete shutdown of body and mind. Pessimistic and with strong views on life, they cannot seem to change what is wrong and remain stuck in trauma.

They will give up, sit back, and let things happen, spiralling into depression, mental paralysis and eventually, suicidal thoughts. They may also turn these experiences outwards and inflict pain on others, even to the point of wanting to commit murder.

Their situation is usually beyond salvage—completely hopeless and full of despair. They are desperate for change, so will actively destroy an unpleasant situation, making it worse to the point of it being unsalvageable. Their pain will cause health to deteriorate to the extreme where they cannot cope with anything, not even themselves. At this point, death seems like the only option.

There are close connections here both with addiction and crime. Others will look on as they descend into alcoholism or drug taking; feeding their habit with criminal activities. Violent crime and sadism without remorse are also indicated here. They possess morbid impulses, which are also destructive in nature and result.

Wherever things are extreme, destructive, and impossible to deal with, the Syphilitic miasm is often the core challenge. Extreme mental issues and terminal dis-ease, as well as dis-eases that affect the skeletal system, are some of its indicators.

The **Tubercular** miasm has a profound effect on respiration and the lungs, although the symptoms will often change and shift location. A person affected by this miasm is frequently self-destructive and would have been often seen as a *problem child* in infancy.

It involves a sense of intense oppression and exploitation with a desire for change, but actions are conducted in such an intense and hectic way that results are rarely achieved. They fear old age and feel they have so little time left—too much to accomplish, so they work at a hectic pace; always rushed and racing against time.

Feeling suffocated and pushed to extremes, they will burn out to the point of total destruction. They throw temper tantrums to get attention and wander from place to place, always moving or relocating themselves with a restless air. They are dissatisfied with life and hate routine which often means they cannot finish things or stick to one task. They are desperate for change and new adventures.

They feel romantically unfulfilled and crave love, but never seem to find it—only to throw it away when they do. Therefore, their heart seems lost and alone.

They are inclined to have affairs and be promiscuous, as well as recurring to self-harming for attention.

Physical symptoms regularly centre around the chest, such as TB, asthma, weak lungs, etc. They may also display symptoms such as bleeding gums, sweating profusely, bloody stools, and diarrhoea.

When it comes to the secondary forms of miasm, we can also connect symptom profiles to the underlying miasmatic issue. For example, the **cancer** miasm presents as a person needing to perform exceedingly well; to live up to very high expectations. They react with a superhuman effort—stretching themselves beyond the limits of their capacity. As they embark on a continuous and prolonged struggle which seems to have no end, they believe failure will result in death and destruction.

The **acute** profile is of extreme threat, where the person will instinctively act in extreme ways— suddenly springing into action, before completely resigning themselves to doing nothing. The **thyroid** miasm presents itself through a competitive attitude, loss and business failure. They experience terrible periods of loss but manage to get through them.

The **ringworm** miasm alternates between periods of struggle with anxiety about success, and periods of despair and giving up. They make a concerted effort but sink down again. The major theme is of unsuccessful efforts; always trying but not succeeding.

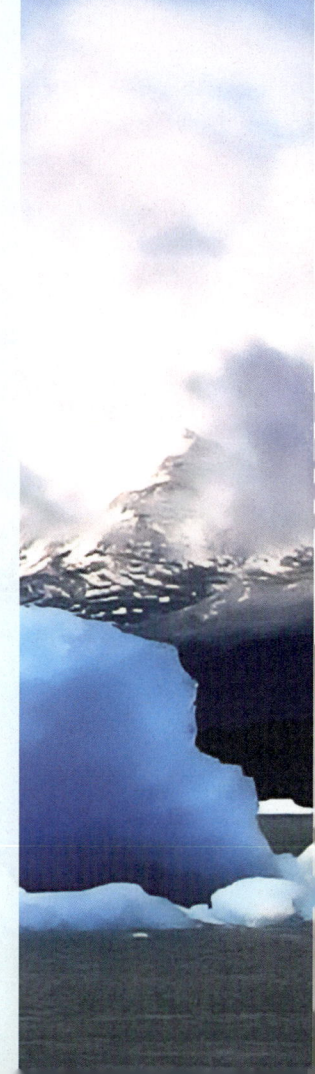

An individual experiencing the **malaria** miasm will experience acute threat that comes in phases, intermingled with feelings of weakness and ineffectiveness. They feel weak and just accept that as inevitable; they resign themselves to bad luck, being hindered, and never achieving anything much at all.

A **leprosy** profile wants to change but experiences intense oppression and hopelessness. They find it difficult to relate to others and feel displaced by others—cast aside and banished from their family or community. They struggle to find their place in the world and always seem unwanted or unable to help, no matter how hard they try.

The **HIV/AIDS** profile is a powerful need to change the world; to break down barriers, stigma and prejudice—often without success. Frequently feeling helpless they can also have a strong desire to keep battling. They will also be very focused on technology, change and development—the evolving roles of women, quality, and social justice.

Finally, the **petrochemical** miasm usually features erratic mood swings, low self-esteem, anxiety and little resistance to stress. Strange, unexpected behaviour is often displayed, along with hormone issues, dis-ease inflicted by action (such as alcohol damage, etc.) and autism.

The miasmatic form of dis-ease is not the actual dis-ease that caused the miasm—a person with the Syphilitic miasm does not have syphilis. Each miasm may, in reality, have very different symptoms to the dis-ease that originally caused it and whilst some indicators may be similar, we must never confuse the miasm with the dis-ease.

When working with therapies such as homoeopathy or Lemurian Celtic Reiki, we often seek to identify the miasm through exploring the client's symptoms. In KRT, we explore their miasmatic experience through the Box Arena environment. Here we interpret imagery, sensation and synaesthesia to identify ancestral miasma.

Within the box, you will experience different elements of dis-ease and trauma that affect the client, whilst influencing their behaviour and choice. Through these experiences, we realise that miasms not only are dis-ease-based but can also be originated by severe, traumatic events/encounters, such as war, natural disasters and cycles of abuse.

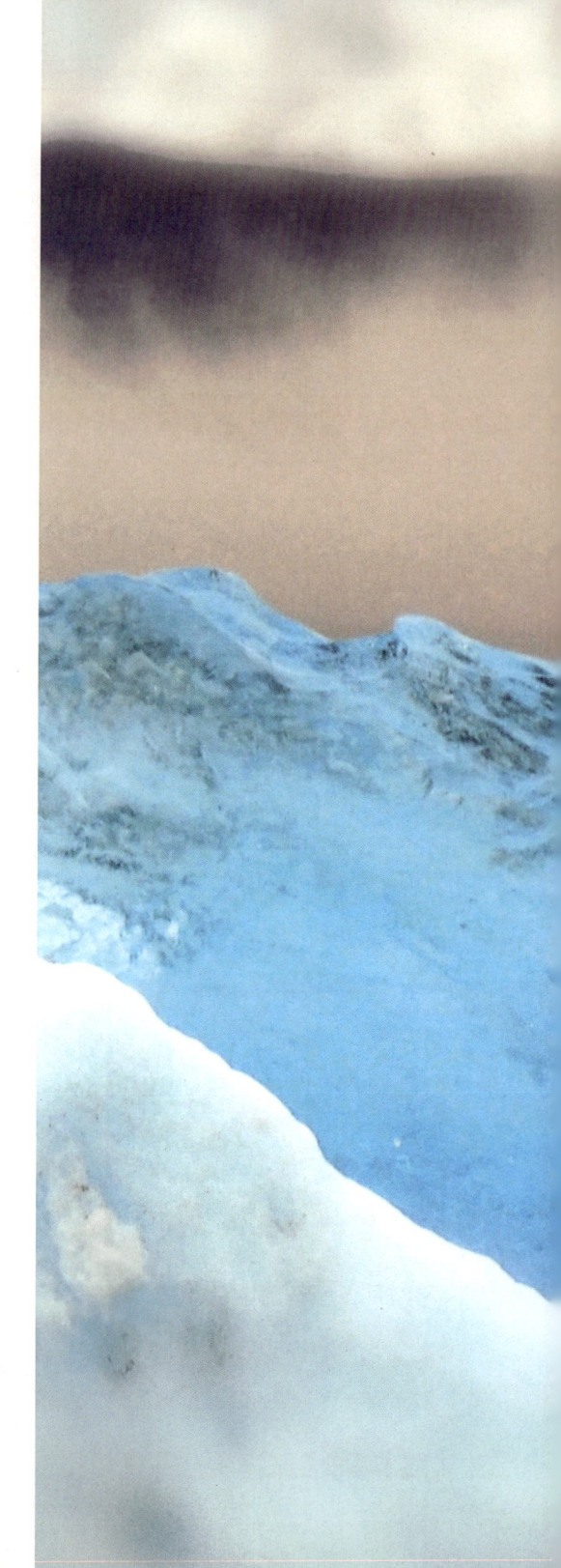

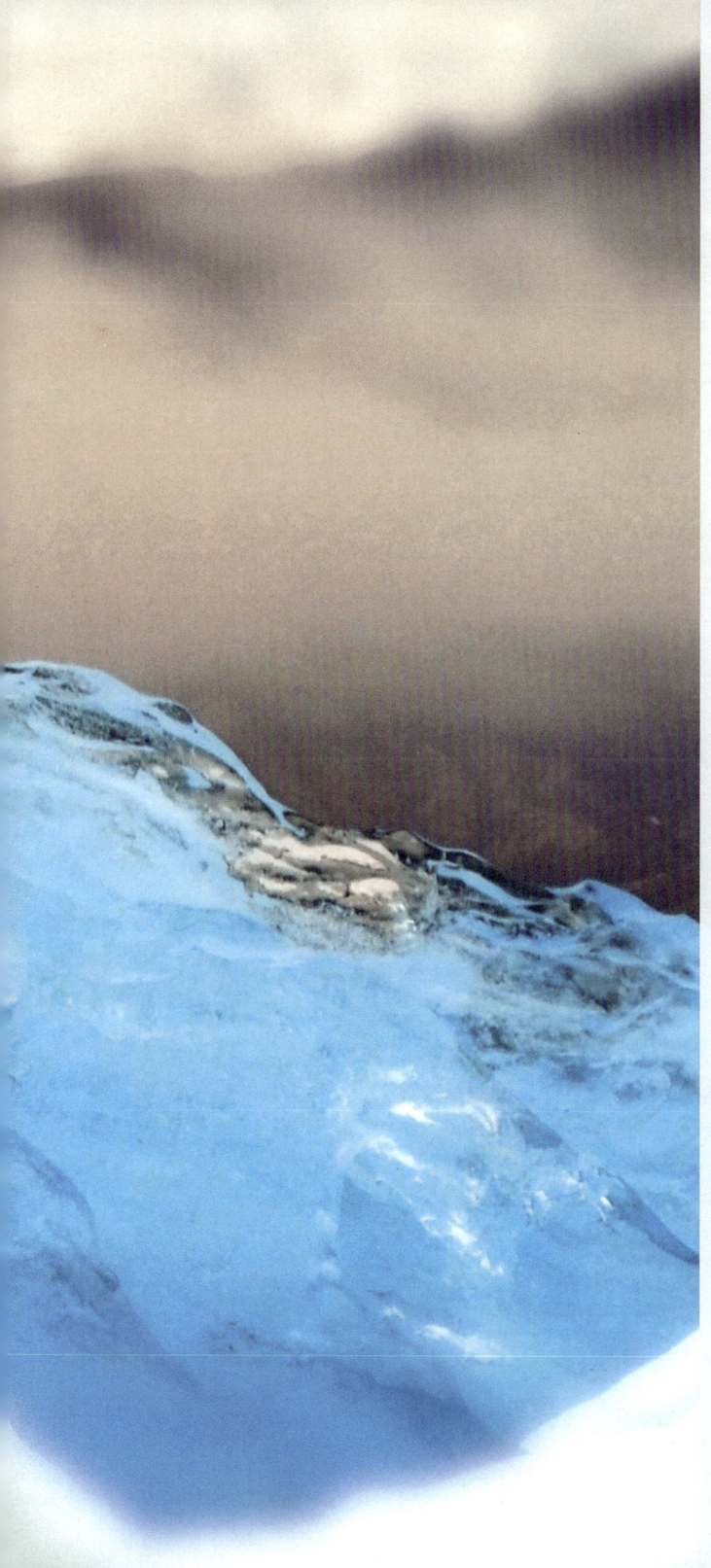

These profoundly traumatic or shocking encounters not only leave an indelible mark on the individual who witnesses them but also affect their children and ancestral line. Therefore, as you treat and clear the vibrational miasma, you are creating a healthier life for your client and those who are yet to come.

For many years, professionals in the field of vibrational therapies have speculated that clearing miasmatic dis-ease can actually heal both directly (the client) and indirectly (the client's family). When we look to the concept of entrainment, we can certainly appreciate how the benefits of treatment could cascade from person to person.

Once your client has experienced the healing effects of a treatment, those with similar miasmatic issues learn how to spontaneously heal themselves, by sensing the change when coming into contact with your client. Of course, when treating clients, any miasmatic connections you share will also initiate a healing reaction within you as well.

Using the foundation treatment method, you will experience a mixture of karmic and miasmatic events, objects and patterns, which you may seek to define or differentiate from each other. However, this is more for the purpose of feedback for your client, rather than having any bearing on your course of treatment (the clearing of the karmic/miasma).

Once, you have calibrated to the Miasmatic KRT Orientation, you will possess a greater sensitivity to miasm-based experiences as well as the nuances in treating these. To the experienced KRT practitioner, karmic patterns and miasmatic vibrations feel very different and have a very different effect on both client and therapist.

Adjusting your treatment method to a miasm-focused method will not only help you fine tune your feedback for the client, but you will also be able to support them better through the healing journey and attain better results from treatment.

Once you have completed the calibration according to the Miasmatic KRT Orientation at least once, adapt your practice method for miasm-specific sense/healing treatments.

Technique:

- Start by standing (or sitting) with your hands on either side of your client's head around the temple area, creating a connection with your client.
- If you wish to do so, ask for higher guidance of some kind to support you during this treatment.
- Now continue by triggering the *Primer* tool.
- After a few minutes, you should begin to feel a really good connection with your client.
- State, internally, that you are conducting a *miasmatic treatment*.
- Now trigger the *Sensing* tool and hold this is one hand (usually your dominant hand), then trigger the *mSense* variant and hold this in the other hand. Wait for the two sensations to balance and then continue.
- Start to move the experience of their auric field through the box, using your hands to decipher the flows/bounce.
- As you locate different dynamics, distortions, and disruptions, constantly ask yourself "What is this?", "How is this affecting my client?", "Where is it from?" and so on. Be aware of any synaesthetic response you attain and use these responses as a *way into* the miasmatic experience (story).
- Once you have exhausted the experience of a miasm, use the *mClearing* until the object is diminished.
- Then, work for a further two-to-three minutes with the *Soothing* and *Sealing*, before venturing on to the next object.
- Once you have completed the main elements of the treatment, work with the *Sealing* for a further five minutes or so.
- Finally, bring your partner fully back into the room.

This slight variation of the treatment, using the mSense adjustment to the Sense tool, will help you differentiate between karma and miasma until you have practised enough to decipher the contrast automatically.

When it comes to the mClearing tool, this slight variation in vibration is adapted to the darker, heavier and more internal/visceral experience that comes with the miasmatic fog. You trigger both this and the mSense tools in exactly the same way as the usual tools, except here you change the name, adding the *m* to the Sense/Clearing tool mantra.

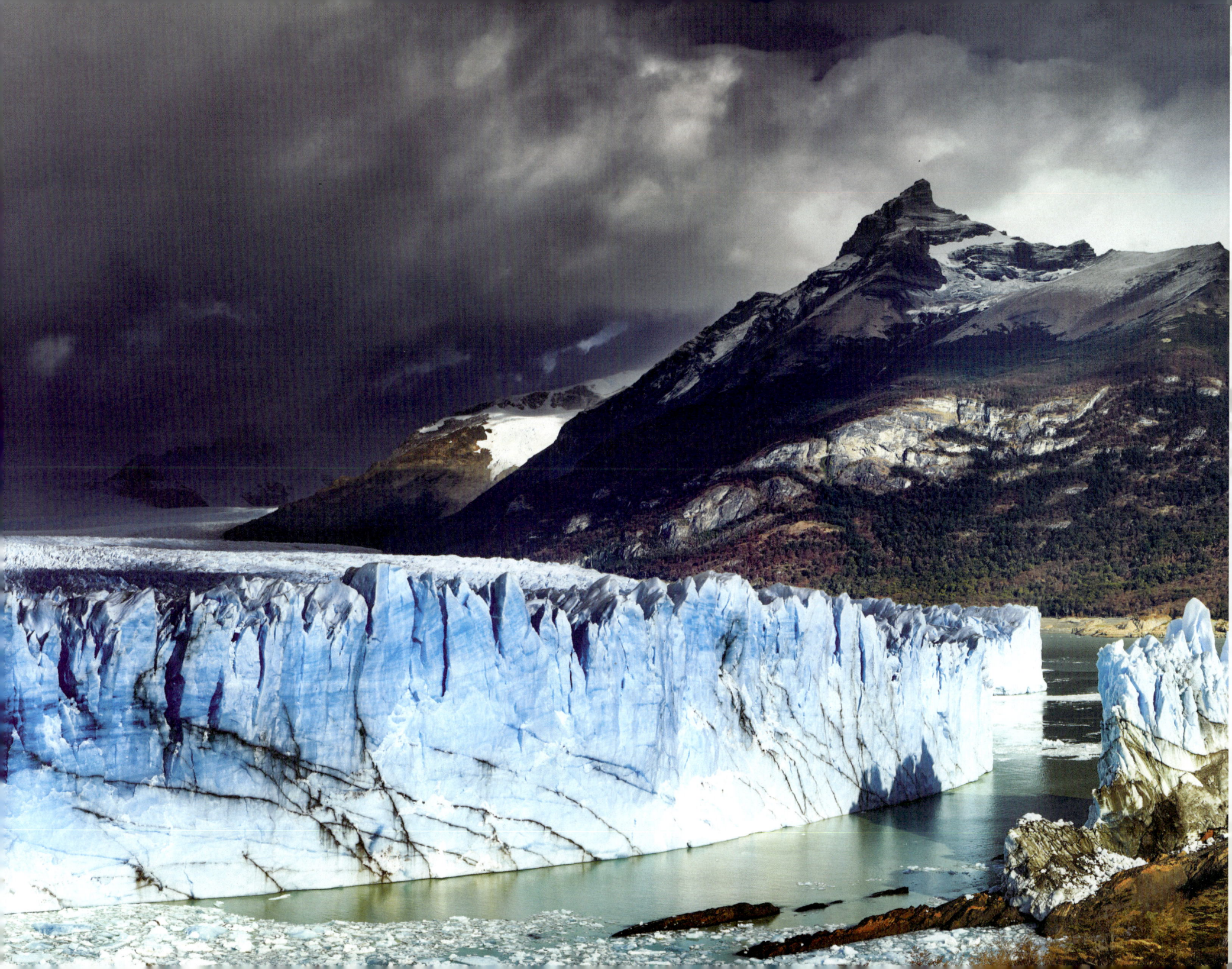

Transpersonal (Holographic) Regression

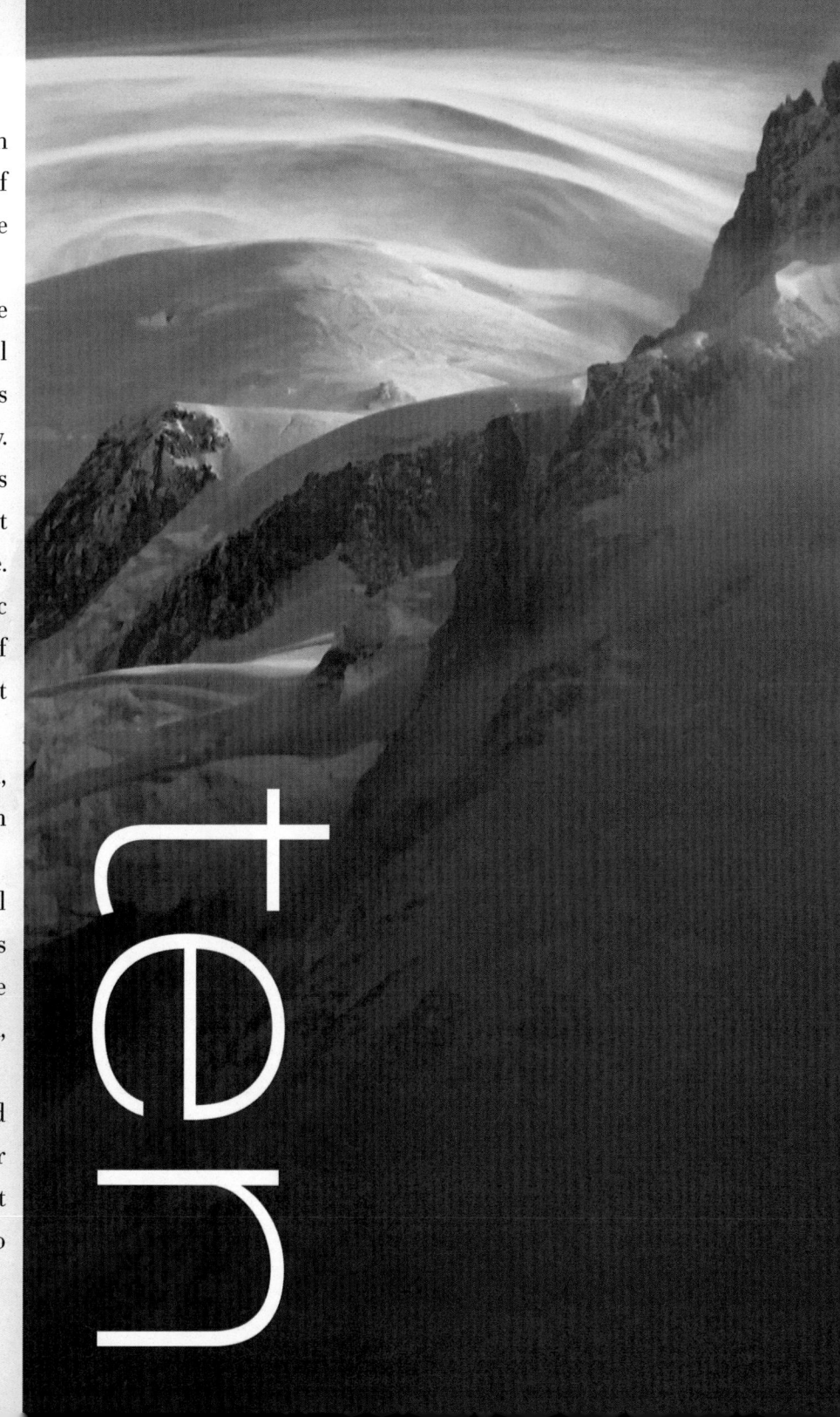

The concept of **subtle memory** is finding growing acceptance as an increasing number of academics and specialists explore the ethos of transpersonal psychology. Stanislav Grof, for example, is leading the way in transpersonal thinking.

Grof believes that every person has access to an indefinable wealth of memories that are not confined to the individual, but to all individuals. This resource of memories could be seen to encompass every experience that has ever been had or will ever be had by everybody.

These experiences form a definitive repository of living memories at a subtle level. These subtle memories are contained within us all at a foundation level, creating holographic pieces of the whole experience.

As we expand from the concept of a soul going on a karmic journey from body to body to the less possessive miasmatic ethos of ancestral heritage, we experience definite shifts in the way we conduct our practice.

Ownership of karma becomes something for families to heal, instead of being some archaic action of a soul that now resides within one person.

Moving onto the transpersonal layer of KRT we arrive at a global form of treatment, where personal responsibility for healing karma is paramount. Each of us is responsible for the whole from our own, unique perspective. Thus, we are each encouraged to act with compassion, behave with dignity, and to give to all.

This in itself is very empowering, because if a problem was caused by somebody else, often they are the one to fix it. When you shift your perspective to understand that you can take responsibility for what happens in your life, you can change it—you reclaim your power to make a difference.

The transpersonal or holographic experience of KRT builds upon the foundation of healing all karma/miasma by defining two points in one's own lifetime and using these to develop a holographic understanding of the dis-ease (and healing) process. These two points are the most significant—birth and death.

The life of a human body begins with the processes of conception and birth, and it ends with the processes of death. In our physical perception, we view our lives as happening between these two points as a series of moments. These moments create what we know as time perception.

However, this time perception is an illusion, because it is merely the interpretation of a series of systematic events, as recognised by our brains. According to the way our brain encodes reality, our birth has already occurred in our perception of time, but our death is still to come.

Though our deaths have yet to be perceived, we know that our deaths exist, albeit in a state of infinite regress— at some point you will come to the end of your life, it is unavoidable, nonetheless this event is based upon an infinite array of choices you have yet to become consciously aware of. Therefore, the circumstances of your own death remain in the realm of possibility, but your death still exists in the universe.

Birth could be viewed as easier to define, because it is part of the individual person's experience, even if this is sub-consciously based. According to Stanislav Grof, the renowned psychotherapist and originator of *Holotropic Breathwork*, the conception/birth process can be divided into four distinct elements:

·   Amniotic Universe (the womb). Blissful feelings of peace and joy, in a healthy womb, which acts as a sanctuary for the new physical life.
·   Cosmic Engulfment (no exit). Contractions begin, accompanied by the unbearable feeling of being stuck with no way of escaping.
·   Death/Rebirth Struggle (second clinical stage of childbirth). Intense struggle for survival, empathy for self as mother and self as child.
·   Death/Rebirth Experience (child is born). Intense, ecstatic feelings of liberation, success and love. Challenges, triumphantly overcome.

These four stages fit very well in the KRT practitioner framework. We can also add a fifth, precursor stage, which is:

·   Dual Awareness (pre-conception and conception). The sperm and the egg awareness. The desperate struggle to create life, followed by the ecstatic rewards of conception.

With these five distinct elements of the conception/birth process, we turn our attention to the death process, which is a far greater challenge to decipher, without much empirical or experiential data about the *death adventure*.

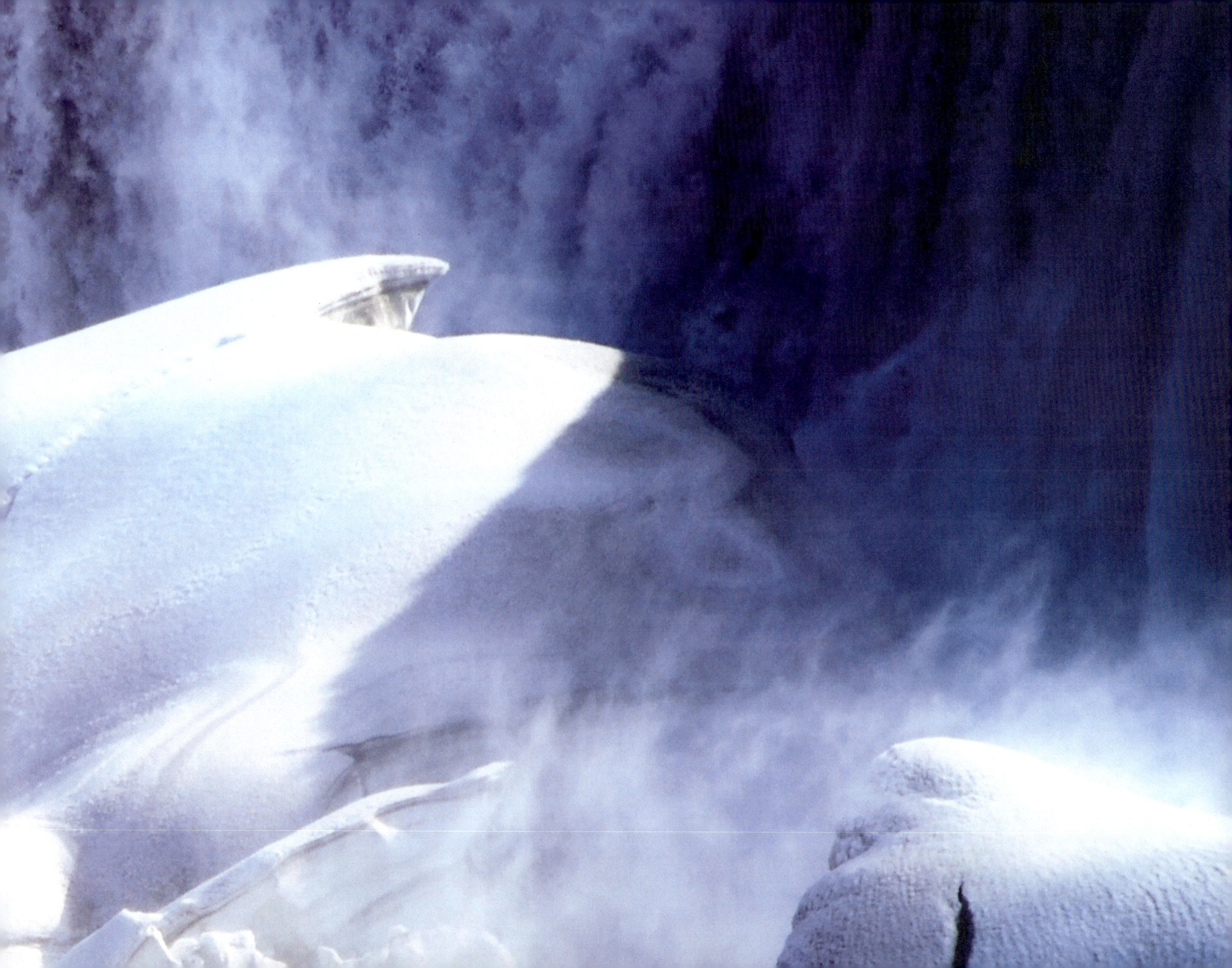

There is speculation that one hundred different stages exist in the death process. Here, one to ten are equivalent to the stages of anaesthesia in surgical procedures. This is, of course, speculation and therefore requires a different and more creative approach.

Let us hypothesise that, at this moment, you are living your life based upon choices that create a specific death adventure process (which is a deep-seated, subconscious decision made at some level of your being). We could say that the effects of this process will be affecting you at this moment because your current situation and circumstances are leading you towards that point in experience.

By adjusting your choices and actions at this point, you start to peruse other choices of death adventure, until you discover the one you would prefer at a conscious level. I believe that all death adventures, although entered into with varying amounts of trepidation and fear, can soon become joyous, blissful adventures.

Nonetheless, the processes of death, as we shall see, play an integral part in the life of a physical being and our choice of death adventure may actually surprise us in the context of KRT.

Now that we have two points of definition—conception/birth and death—we have the *parameters of interaction*, by which we can create a treatment. By nature, professional KRT treatments are holographic in design.

A hologram occurs when a laser (split into two separate beams) is focused on a three-dimensional object. This creates interactions between the two beams that reflect onto a holographic plate. The plate is formed of many cells, each of which records the information of the entire laser interaction.

Thus, the plate offers in two dimensions, the illusion of the original, three-dimensional object. This is remarkable, as any single cell contains the information for the whole, viewed from the cell's perspective. (It is important to remember perspective in this philosophy because if you were to cut the holographic plate in half, only the remaining half of the object would be visible on the plate, rather than the whole object only smaller. This is because the whole is seen from the perspective of each cell, instead of from an overview perspective.)

So, the five stages of birth for each individual, once interacting with their death adventure, create the illusion of life. Every moment of our experience is a holographic combination of the contraction into physical form (conception/birth) and the expansion into energy (death). The juxtaposition of these two polar opposites acts as the interaction for our holographic life and form the choices that we filter every experience through.

And whilst this may seem to be similar to the idea of fate, here we can see the distinction between traditional and KRT perspectives. Your birth is at some level a static event, experienced in the past and it is often presumed that our death is equally set in stone. However, in KRT practice we recognise the idea that we have infinite possibilities of experience that stem from the death adventure. We all die, but how we die is a subliminal choice that changes upon our perception at the moment.

Every interaction creates a moment that we perceive via sensory information, filter and consciously experience as part of life. Also, these interactions contain the information of the whole, viewed from that perspective. This means that at any given point in our lives, we can not only choose what to experience but also how to alter the next moment to a consciously decided possibility, based on an awareness of our whole potential life. This, in turn, means that we actively shape, not only our perception of life but also the physical reality we encounter as part of the perceived, linear journey.

To further unravel this multifaceted concept of shifting goal posts, possibilities, potential experiences, choices and perspective, let us examine the processes and ideas of the holographic life at a deeper level. Starting with the journey of conception and birth, followed by the death adventure, and finally the holographic interactions of both points.

The Stages of Conception and Birth

When in a state of deep hypnotic trance, meditation, or even some forms of psychotropic state, it is possible to revisit times throughout our lives before birth and even prior to conception. Those who have regressed back to these ancient times in their physical existence often report information, which is then verified by the person's mother.

This may take the form of some trauma faced whilst in the womb, strangulation by the umbilical cord, forceps used during the birthing process, or caesarean section. Holotropic breathwork practitioners and hypnotherapists offer feedback gleaned from thousands of people over many years.

This data consistently displays a correlation between altered state experience and parental verification, even when the subject had no prior knowledge of the circumstances of their birth.

By gaining a conscious awareness of their own conception and birth process, a person often realises the various effects these early times have throughout their life. In KRT, it also enables you to become aware of your own facets in relation to the contractive dynamics you face and can then treat.

Each of the five stages can create parameters that stay with a person their whole life, contained in the holographic interactions that act as filters of our experience. Thus, by examining these five stages, we can locate and target areas of possible interest and treatment.

Dual Awareness

The dual awareness stage is one of immense struggle and overwhelming joy. The majority of sperm and eggs never come to fruition in a physical sense, even though every sperm and egg ever created has the potential to become a living being. The intense challenge that faces each are usually too much for all but a minute few and this inconceivable effort is often played out in adult life, especially in the areas of work or relationships. We forget the absolute joy as sperm and egg conceive new life and focus on the exhaustive journey to reach that moment.

Conversely, by reliving that struggle in therapy a client can be directed to focus on the extremely high levels of motivation, the fighting spirit of their first ever challenge—the challenge that made them a complete success before they were even born! As they reach the point of conception, a person can become overwhelmed with joy, frequently recognising the event as the most profound and rapturous occasion in their life.

We could view this stage with the analogy of a marathon runner, who spends months training in readiness for their physical and psychological ordeal. They find the strength, stamina, and willpower to complete their challenge, but upon completion of the marathon, all they remember is the pain and torment of the actual running—the high of the endorphins and the joy of achieving their goal is lost in the muscle cramps and burning lungs.

Therapeutically, we are simply asking the runner to remember the factors that enabled them to succeed and the joy of the destination. Any form of trauma in this stage of life is known in KRT terms as Duality Holographic Trauma (DHT).

Amniotic Universe

In the majority of cases, our first nine months of life, cosseted away in the safety of the womb, is a tranquil and blissful time. All we know is warmth and comfort in our dark, all-encompassing sanctuary.

Our reward for such an enormous achievement is a seemingly endless time of nurture and connection, where our every whim is catered for by our mother's body. The first thing we know on Earth is a completely engulfing *amniotic universe* – it is all there is, and we cannot use words to describe how wonderful it is.

However, there are some exceptions to this seemingly eternal realm of peace and love. A foetus whose mother smokes, drinks, takes drugs, or in some other way intoxicates her body will often experience trauma or some other form of reaction. Likewise, physical, emotional, or psychological trauma to the mother will also affect the unborn child. Disease, lack of nutrition and environmental factors may also play a part in disrupting the bliss state.

These and other factors may manifest in the adult person as an inability to experience comfort, joy, happiness, relaxation, and so on. In some cases, they may even become fearful of womb-like environments, developing triggers to claustrophobia or sleep disorders. An inability to be happy, overwork, stress, etc., can all be perceivable signals of Holographic Womb Trauma (HWT).

Cosmic Engulfment

The first clinical stage of childbirth, when the contractions begin, literally gives us our concept of contraction into life. As the mother prepares to give birth, her body begins to repel

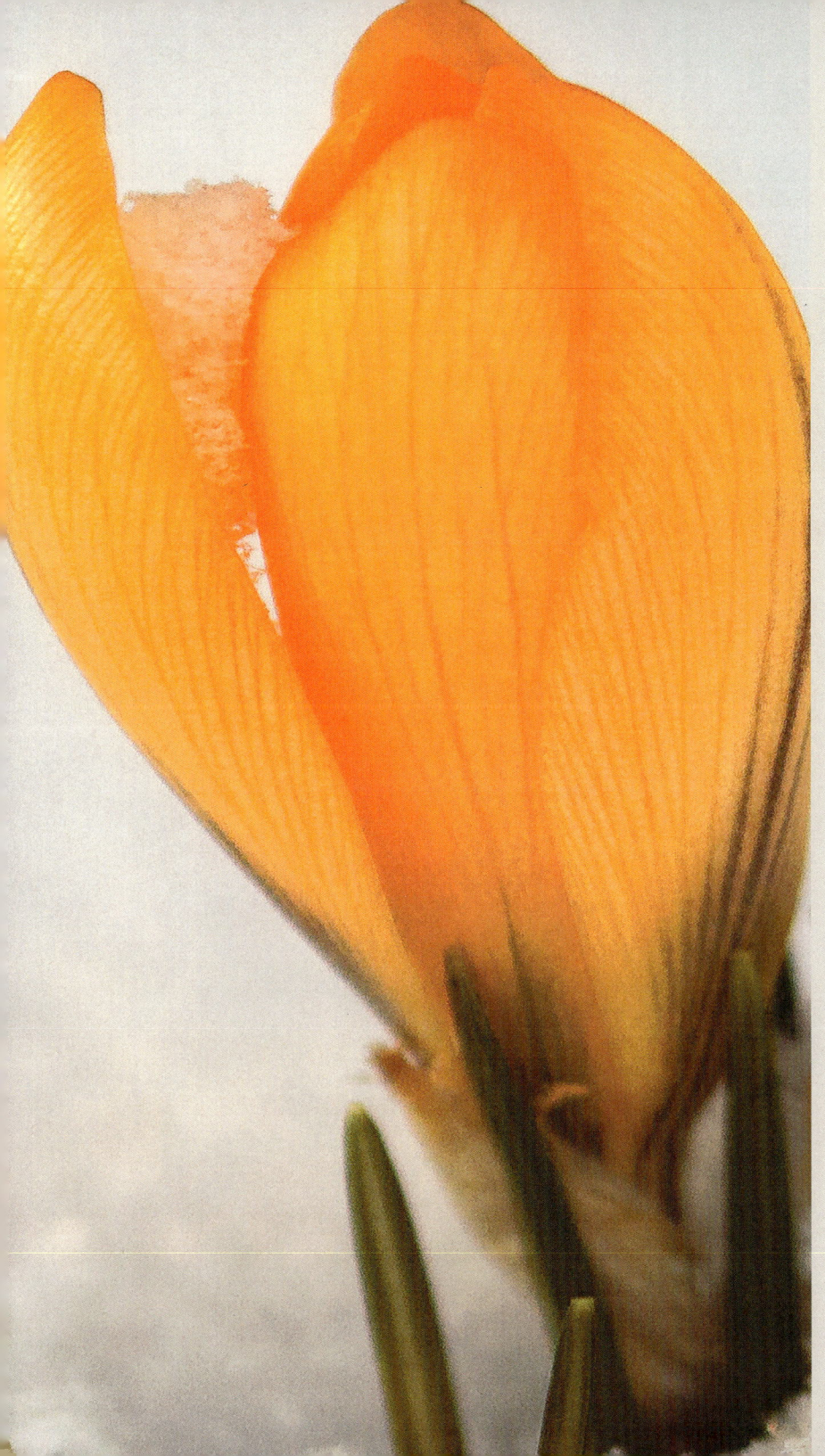

the child, literally creating a toxic, deadly environment from which the baby must escape. For a while, however, there is no escape, no clear way out of the womb, where the foetus has spent a blissful eternity. It is almost an experience of being casted out from paradise, or a descent into hell.

Everything we have ever known crumbles around us and, for the first time, death becomes a very real possibility. We experience our own death at a conscious level, and the holographic interactions between birth and death become fully-realised.

As the child senses her dilemma, she recognises trauma, possibly for the first time. Her situation of being completely stuck, without any hope of escape, may cause her to despair. This stage of the birthing process may cause her to experience trauma and abuse her entire life. Sadness, fear, hate, dis-ease, feeling unloved or uncared for, loneliness and depression can all be linked to this stage of birth; Clinical Stage One Holographic Trauma (CS₁HT).

Death/Rebirth Struggle

In the second clinical stage of childbirth, a real sense of life, death and rebirth develops as the baby recreates his dual-awareness struggle to survive. Not only is there an epic journey involved as the birth canal opens and the child begins to make his way into the world, but he also experiences a strange duality of self. Identifying both as a unique and distinct individual and with his mother, he becomes the abused and the abuser. He can empathise with both sides of the dynamic and understands his situation as a whole.

As his intense struggle for survival continues, the baby may come into contact with bodily fluids, waste products, such as urine or faeces, as well as blood, etc. This visceral, overwhelming battle to survive, is a test for the child on every level, as he not only fights for life, but also for his own identity and individuality.

This stage can be seen as a progression from the last stage—a realisation of why this situation is occurring. As the death/rebirth struggle continues, the child understands the greater reasons behind his challenge and at the same time is still partaking in the challenge. Here, the child feels abused, yet understands why he is being abused; he feels pain and torment but realises the greater purpose of the trials he is enduring.

The Clinical Stage Two Holographic Trauma (CS2HT) can result in the want to be abused or hurt in some way, such as people who are bullied or those who want to experience S&M practices, etc.

Obsessive behaviour, particularly to do with cleanliness, infection, waste products, etc., can also be a result of the holographic interactions of this stage. If strangulation by the cord, breach birth or other incident occurs, it is at this particular stage that the holographic interactions will be most prevalent.

Death/Rebirth Experience

As the child is born, she announces to the world her arrival with a defiant, yet joyful scream. This state is a passing through death to be reborn and is accompanied by integral, ecstatic feelings of liberation and success. The challenge of facing one's own death is completed, and a new life begins, accompanied by the vast rewards of experience in the physical world.

It is at this point the adventure begins for the child; every smile or laugh, every tear or heartbreak is a blissful experience that can only be really appreciated in physical form. Our universal self knows all these emotions and sensations, it understands/knows the reasons for them in a balanced and complete way, yet to experience them anew via the illusion of separateness is what enables the universe to know the joy and pain it is capable of.

In this rewarding and triumphant stage of birth, Rebirth Holographic Traumas (RHT) occur when the opportunity for success is taken away from the child, for example in cases of caesarean section, or when forceps are used. In these instances, a person may often repeat struggles for survival or success, without ever reaping the rewards—choosing to fail at the last minute, when a happy end is in sight.

The five stages of conception/birth discussed here act as a framework that enables us to pinpoint areas of trauma in a client's life (from our own perspective). For, not only do Holographic Traumas become apparent when compared with birth processes, but we also tend to cycle our daily life circumstances and situations according to these stages.

For instance, a person may work hard for something in their life, struggling to achieve until they get to the state where they feel content/safe (dual awareness). They then coast along in this state, choosing not to change or deviate from their comfort zone (amniotic universe). Eventually, without change on a voluntary level, the circumstances will change, sometimes creating drastic, sometimes deeply traumatic change (cosmic engulfment).

This contraction into trauma is soon after accompanied by an understanding of why these changes have taken place and even empathy for the processes at work (death/rebirth struggle). Finally, a re-expansion into bliss or rebirth into a potentially 'better' or more successful life situation occurs (Death/Rebirth Experience).

Of course, in this process, a person may encounter issues and challenges that relate either to Holographic Traumas of different stages in the conception/ birth processes, or incongruous interactions with the death adventure, which creates the second factor of the holographic interaction process.

As a KRT practitioner, the initial step would be to locate and treat holographic trauma at conception or birth and then adjust the death adventure to a more conducive interaction state. Firstly, before we examine the procedures for this, let us turn our attention to the death adventure and what we mean by this term.

The Death Adventure

The thought of death is something that terrifies a lot of people because it is beyond anything we can understand or comprehend. Many philosophical or theological debates centre around what happens when we die, it has been the subject of many scientific studies and is something that we all have ideas or opinions on. Death also remains the one certainty for all living things, which is why we often look to our inevitable death with a sense of dread.

To a certain extent, fear of the unknown is hardwired into the human psyche, though how we experience and deal with that fear is a matter of individual choice. Some people are paralysed by it, some revel in it; some take action to overcome their fears, whilst others are buried underneath them. It seems only natural, therefore that we may be slightly anxious about death, which is after all, the great unknown.

There are those who attempt to come to terms with the inevitable death of the physical body by looking to energy, to the soul, whilst others resign themselves to having as much joy, happiness and fun in life as possible, just in case that is all there is!

In his book, *The Endorphin Effect*, William Bloom discusses the ability of every single living cell to produce the pleasure-giving neurochemical, encephalin (endorphins). Bloom explains his belief that we live in an ultimately benevolent universe, where every living creature from the most advanced primates and cetaceans to the single-celled amoeba will die in a pleasure-soaked wave of absolute bliss and comfort.

This is because every part of our physical being will explode with encephalin as we reach a certain point in the death process. Our last pieces of consciousness on Earth will be joyous moments of rapture, without pain or remorse.

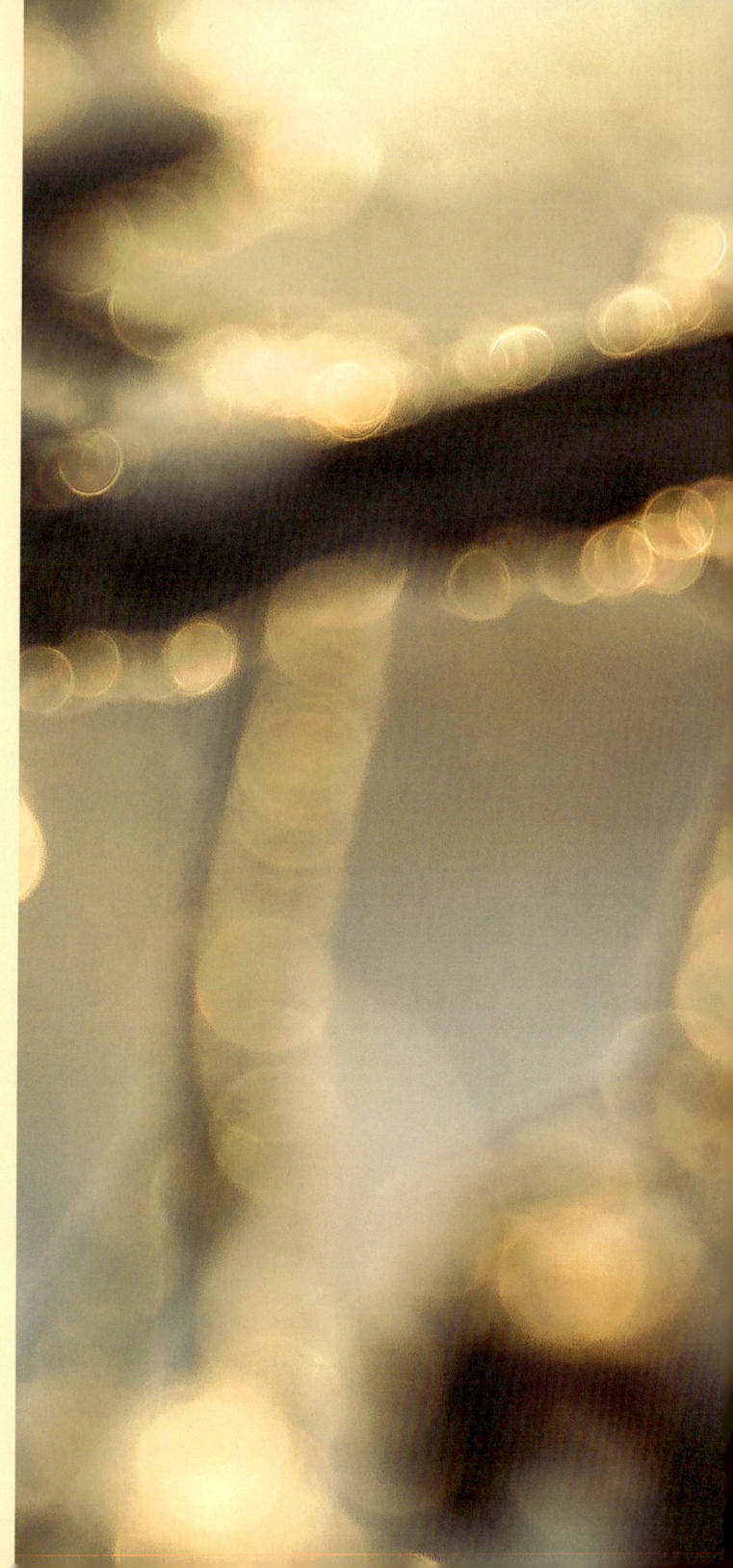

In a KRT sense, every moment of life is filled with joy and bliss, even our darkest experiences. Once you have connected to a state of expansion and have learnt the ability to retain this connection, even when in the pits of despair, you can still know joy and happiness. It seems, therefore that your last moments in life should be no exception.

Actually, in KRT terms, the death process is an adventure, a journey into the unknown, filled with unexpected twists and turns, and new perspectives, where joyous secrets are revealed.

The realisation of your own perfection and connection to the physical world as an enlightened being can often enable you to understand the full workings of solidity and how the physical body's death is merely another experience to be cherished and experienced to the full.

In fact, the release of our integral ties to the physical and the body, liberate us to the point of actively participating in our death adventure, without fear or trepidation. It is something to look forward to, to experience in every moment as holographic interactions, it is a part of us, as integral as our birth and as every moment we perceive in life.

As an essential part of the physical body, our consciousness is a little harder to reconcile in this process, suffice it to say that we will more than likely experience the amazing wonder of complete encephalin saturation and the knowledge that our consciousness has touched and influenced many—just as they have done, us.

Of course, when discussing the death adventure as part of our holographic interactions, we avoid speculation of the sensations and experience itself and focus more on how the death adventure interacts with our conception/birth to create our lives. You see, this is not just a question of the two interactions influencing our lives, the death/birth holography actually creates lives.

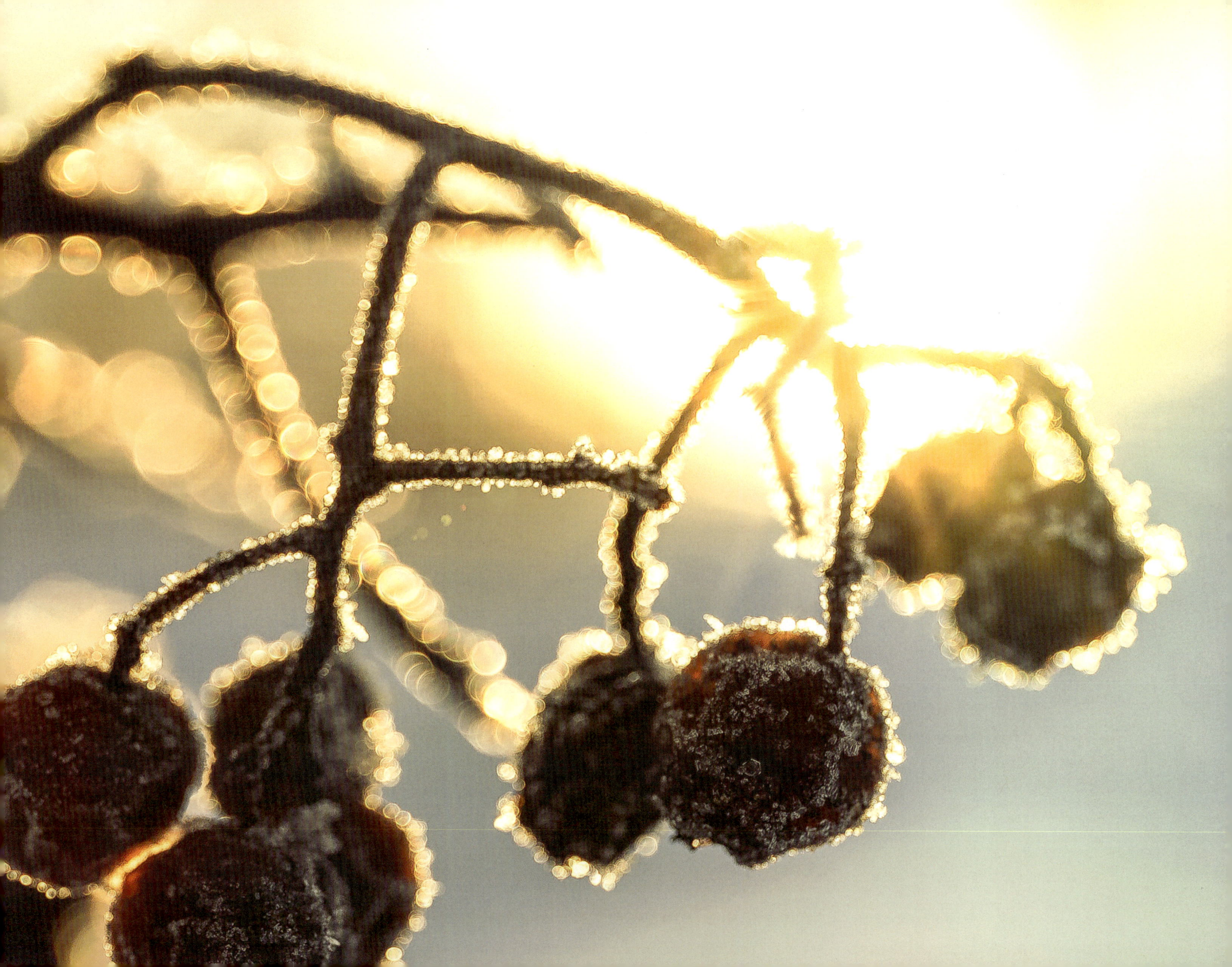

Each birth is a contraction of light into physicality, whilst each death is an expansion of physicality into light. These contractions and expansions interact to form holographic illusions of life in which the universe is perceived from a point of contraction or expansion, depending on what each consciousness tends to focus upon.

Each and every situation that we encounter has both contraction and expansion as an integral part of the whole. Our conscious experience, though, will only focus on one or the other depending on your habitual response or conscious intervention. In other words, if you are consciously experiencing an event in space and time from an expansive point of view, you will completely filter out all contractive elements of the interaction.

A further point to include here is that, despite a balanced and equal level of interaction exists between birth and death, issues in the five stages of the birth process may create a bias towards contraction. Whilst our fear of death, and an unwillingness to embrace the expansive processes of death, may impede our expansion.

Thus, healing of conception/birth traumas combined with the realignment of the death adventure readdresses the bias of the conscious mind rather than altering the equilibrium of the death/birth interactions, which always remain in balance.

Hence, the main focus when working with the death adventure and forming a realignment of the holographic interactions (choosing other potential points of interaction) is not about deciding *how you are going to die*. It is about choosing *how you are going to live* in relation to the interactions that shape the hologram your senses tell you is your life.

You are, therefore, not flicking through some great *100 Great Ways to Die!* catalogue—you are solely focusing on the effects of change in your interactions. As the holographic illusion makes expansion easier, you know you are aligning to a more conducive death adventure in relation to your conception/birth.

Eventually, an ongoing process of refinement, healing, and alignment will enable you to smooth your daily life into a fine-tuned state of expansion, full of joy and bliss in each moment, regardless of the challenges you face.

Holographic Life Interactions

Every moment of your life is filled with every moment of your life. A peculiar statement, yet in every single moment we encounter, we are actually experiencing every moment that exists potentially. The only reason we do not perceive life in this way is that our consciousness focuses solely on certain aspects of the single moment.

This is rather like being presented with a large plate of food; you do not consume the entire meal in one mouthful. Instead, you consciously eat small quantities at a time, taking a while to chew and swallow before the next.

How we decide what aspects of our encounters we choose depends on the filters consciousness is employing, the memories that are shaping present perception, and what parameters the consciousness believes to be worthy of focus (its reality). Thus, any aspects of a moment that are deemed to be irrelevant by the current filters will be deleted, distorted or generalised, whilst the sensory information that makes it through the filtration process is then shaped and presented according to accessible memory and the preferred version of reality.

By understanding that the holographic nature of our experiences contain far more than we perceive consciously, we enable the restructuring of how we process sensory data to encompass elements of information we choose with volition, instead of being at the mercy of data that is supplied through habitual and learnt responses, or subliminal suggestion.

In other words, most people believe they have their own mind, but they are merely doing what they have learnt to do and thinking how they are told people should, or should not, think. By understanding there is more to life and death than just a straight line of existence between the two, we can break free of simple mimicry and begin to form new connections.

Now, whilst we can create minimal expansion in our consciousness and how much data we can process at any given moment, the notion of changing our perspective is not to *fit more in* (take bigger mouthfuls from our plate), it is to alter what we focus on (choose what type of food to take next.)

With this methodology, we can break old cycles, change our focus from contraction to expansion, create new emotional attachments to thought patterns, become more expanded in perception and the way we sense the physical world, and myriad other things that increase our potential for happiness and joy.

So with this in mind, take some time to visualise two points in your perception. One is your conception/birth; the other, your death. These two points contract into the physical world and expand into light, respectively. Where they interact with the universe (at all points of your perspective), they create your life in infinite possibility.

Your brain filters out the majority of this information and pays conscious attention to what is left, ready to process into memory. In most cases, your brain will constantly be filtering out anything it does not perceive as the *present* moment (the next moment in time); and whilst you may actually be within reach of infinite connection, you will often habitually limit your attention to the boundaries of linear time and space.

KRT Treatment of the Holographic Self

With this understanding of our intent in a Karmic Regression Therapy context, let us now turn our attention to the actual treatment of the holographic self, initially from the point of view of the healing of our conception/birth perspective and then from the alignment of the death adventure style of treatment.

These two styles of treatment can be used separately, although it is recommended to use the Birth Journey first, followed by the Death Adventure Alignment in the subsequent treatment session.

The Birth Journey

The Birth Journey is a mixture of treatment, guided meditation and energy orientation, which centres around the treatment of your perspective of conception and birth. As you treat your own five stages of conception/birth, your client will reflect challenges and issues from their own experience. This synthesis can be augmented with other essences, as required, to completely fulfil the needs of the treatment.

There are three main regions of the treatment, which are:

- Guided journey through the conception and birth process.
- Essence connection to enhance the journey.
- Energy orientation to the point where your five stages are treated from your current perspective.

Begin with your client sitting or lying down in a comfortable position, with all the usual, preferred sensory enhancements of the treatment environment in place (oil/incense, candles, music, etc.). Then, begin a guided journey that will last the whole treatment through. After an initial introduction, it will become an intermittent narration to which you will return every 5-10 minutes or so.

Start the guided instruction by focusing on breathing, then relaxing all the main regions of the body, starting with the feet and working up to the head area (toes, heels, knees, hips, and so on). Return to breathing and count down from 10-1. Use the under/over verse here, for example, "With every number, you feel yourself going deeper into trance," or "You could, if you wanted to, go into the deepest trance you have ever known!"

Regress through time, flying through the sky, drifting in space, etc., to the point just before conception and experience this. Once conception has taken place, move through the next four stages. Ask your client to remember the details, but keep asserting that they are feeling safe, secure and calm.

Trigger *Arena* and initiate the treatment steps before each new section of the guided meditation, as detailed below. When the treatment is complete bring the client back into the room and, after a few moments to collect themselves, ask for feedback. After your client has gone, make some notes on your own experiences of the treatment.

Technique:

- Make your client comfortable in the sitting or lying down position.
- When ready, begin the Guided Journey introduction and make head connection to your client.
- Begin a *Birth Journey* treatment.
- Focus on breathing for three breaths.

- Starting at the feet, work on relaxing each main area of the body up to the head.
- Focus on breathing again.
- Using hypnotic language count down from ten to one.
- Trigger *Arena.*
- Experience the sensation of the treatment commencing.
- Trigger *Primer.*
- Travel back through time to the point just before conception and experience this until conception is complete.
- Trigger *Sensing.*
- Begin to move hand positions/gestures and work around client's body, using *Clearing* and *Soothing.*
- (Amniotic Universe) Move forward to time in the womb, and include any significant events that arose from time spent here—experience the perspective change.
- (Cosmic Engulfment) Continue onwards to the first stage of childbirth, remembering to take your client into third person mode if they feel anxious at any time – experience the changes in perspective once again.
- (Death/Rebirth Struggle) Now move on to the second stage of childbirth and notice perspective change—continue to move around client and intuitively change hand positions/movements.
- (Death/Rebirth Experience) Finally come to the moment of birth and the joyous, liberating feeling that heralds the start of a new life—return to client's head area.
- Trigger *Sealing.*
- Disconnect from your client's head and bring them back into the room by counting up from one to ten.
- Gain feedback and make notes.

Death Adventure Alignment

In this next treatment routine, you will be connecting to and adjusting the holographic interactions between conception/birth and death. This does not mean actually working with the death adventure itself, but experiencing how this affects your perspective when interacting with the birth experiences.

By adjusting the interactions, you will discover aspects that are conducive to a conscious connection to the expansion elements. Therefore, any habitual filtration of perception that favours contraction in consciousness will become less likely to achieve conscious focus.

We could view this as a way of creating a greater conscious focus on the expansion process (which is usually subconscious) as opposed to contraction (mostly conscious). In twenty-first-century society, we tend to look for the answers in the physical—our scientifically-led attitudes have a certain amount of bias towards the *real world*, with answers in what we can perceive using the five senses or technology based on the perspective of those senses.

Focusing on the act of expansion and by creating interactions with patterns of expansion that an individual can recognise, the conscious becomes distracted by the subtle senses (Living Matrix). With regular exposure to these specific patterns, the conscious mind learns how to recognise sensory data from beyond the physical and our state of expansion begins.

At this point, we start exploring our expansion as well as our contraction. In many cases, with experience, we start looking to expansion more than contraction. In these instances, bliss becomes the force of greater connectivity in our psyche.

This denotes that our intent in any treatment featuring the death adventure is one of connectivity. We are looking to find interactions where the conscious mind is distracted by the expansion processes, rather than habitual contraction.

This technique is one that you can refine over time to make your own—an intuitive, interactive, and creative process where you experience contrasting perspectives and alter them according to the way you feel and understand as appropriate.

When a potential future is discovered and connected to, it becomes physical reality and the following holographic moment will usually manifest as some form of beautiful sensory experience or epiphany.

Technique:

· Once your client is comfortable in the seated or lying down position, you can begin.
· Trigger *Arena*.
· Begin a Death Adventure Alignment treatment.

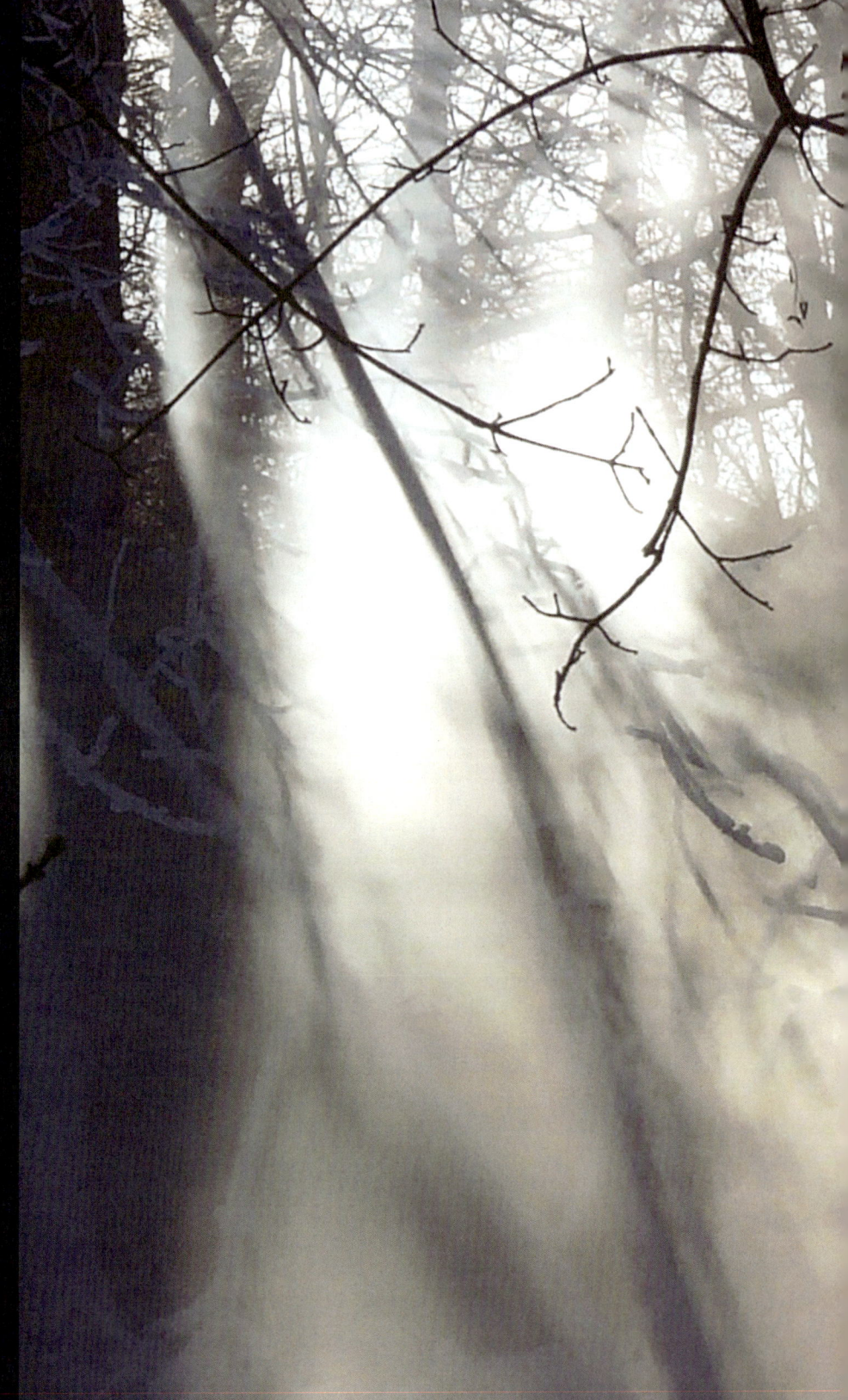

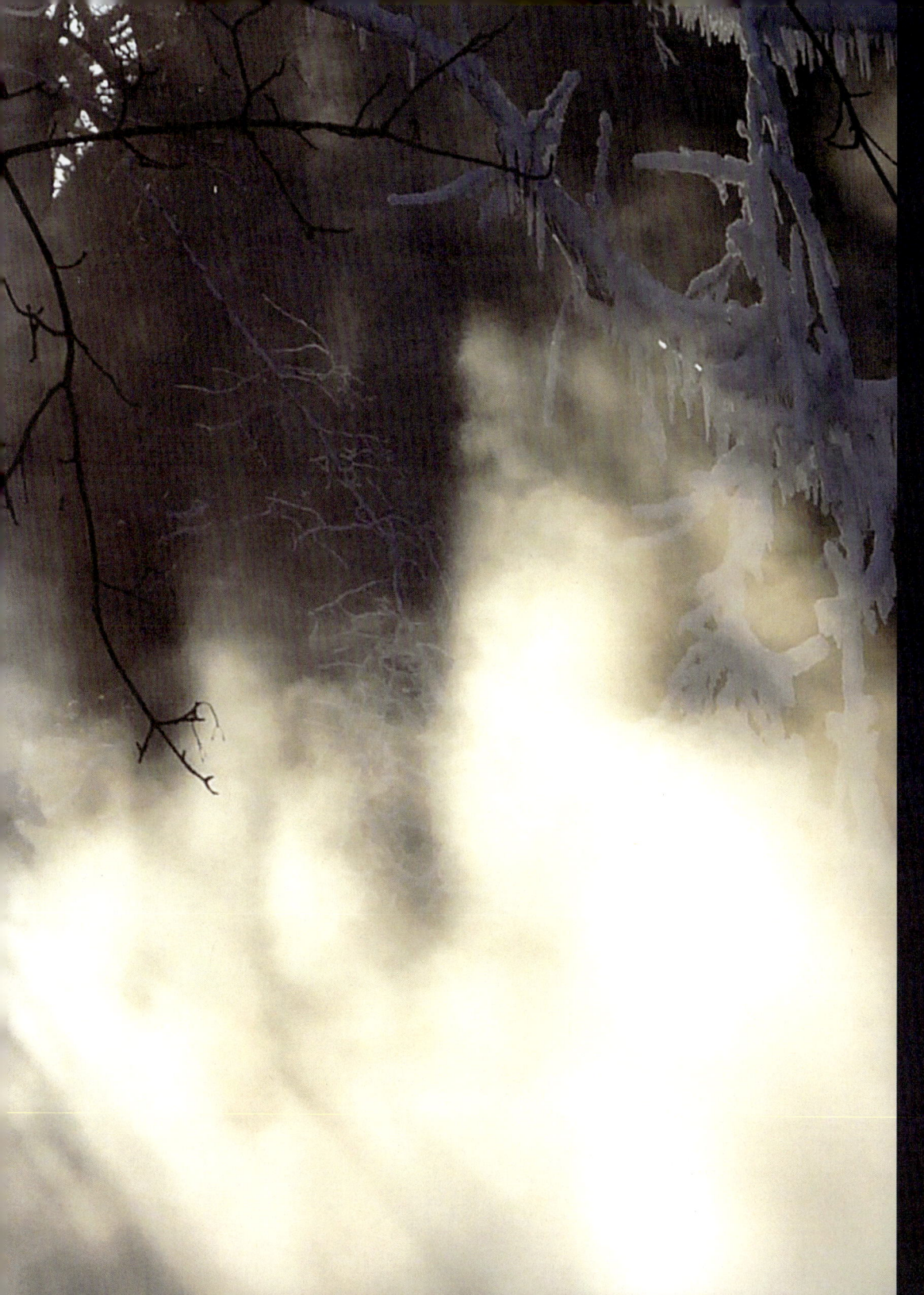

- Trigger *Primer*.
- Make a head connection to your client.
- Trigger *Sensing*.
- Feel the holographic interactions taking place in your consciousness, becoming increasingly aware of contractive and expansive responses, monitoring to which of these you feel more attracted.
- Start to work through intuitive hand positions or gestures on your client; use the *Clearing* and *Soothing* essences.
- Once you have a good sense of the interactions, start to locate the processes of *skimming* or *flipping*, as you experience infinite realities and potential futures in synaesthetic form.
- You may experience this process speeding up or become more like a pulse between two/three different states. Once the final state is found, there will be an almighty shift that changes your perspective.
- Work through the treatment, as you wish, monitoring the vibrations and changes in state—be aware if there is a resistance or wanting to return to old states and reaffirm *Clearing*.
- Once you feel the treatment perspective waning or the session time is up, finish with *Sealing*.
- Bring your client back into the room and discuss their experience—be sure to make notes of your own afterwards.

Viridian Regression

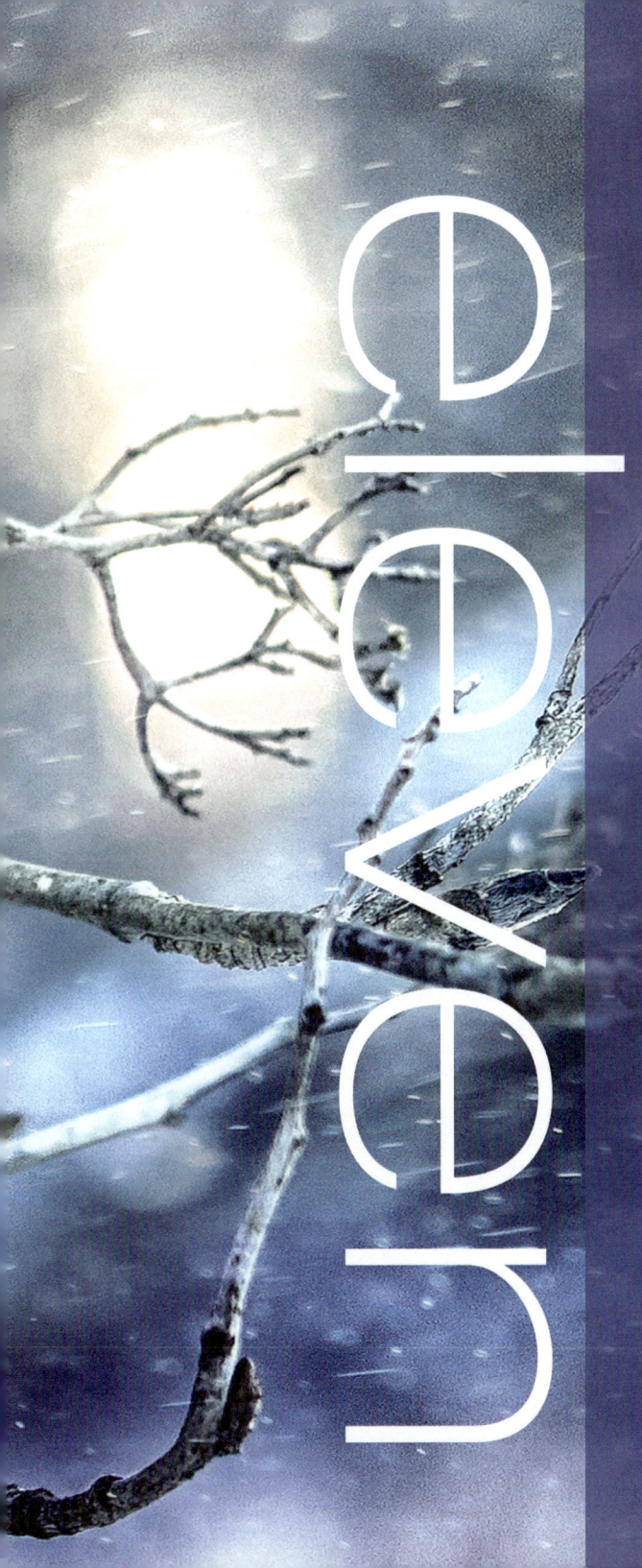

vKRT is the most advanced form of regression therapy we have explored in this practitioner training experience.

The Viridian philosophy, when applied to our existing ethos completely changes how we view time and the experience of time from our professional perspective.

Karma, miasma, birth, and death shift into a very different perspective when you remove time from the equation. In many ways, the foundations of our therapy and the traditions they are built upon are based on time (and separated by it). When you take away time from KRT, you liberate yourself from all the limitations and dogma that come with the temporal experience of life.

At its most simplified, the Viridian philosophy defines several points of consciousness—Potential, I-Self and Viridian State (V-State). These are the infinite array of potential experiences you can have in any given moment; the perspective or self you are experiencing now and the most profound and perfect (best) version of your life/self.

Without time, our birth and death exist in every moment, as does everything in-between—everything we remember and everything we hope for. The difference is that everything we remember is not actually part of our experience, other than the way it is presented to us by our distorted memories. What we hope for consists of anything that is possible for us to experience within a never-ending array of iterations.

Through the I-Self, we can shift into V-State and invoke our greatest vision for life. However, if we do not actively do this, we slip into E-State—Everything Else that could happen and will... without Volition. The polarity between our V and our E is what balances and creates the I.

As our V-State is always filtered through the I-Self, learning how to truly know V-State can be almost impossible; so we use proxies to hold the vision for us and then work with these proxies to develop a greater awareness of when we exist in E and how to voyage into V.

These proxies are physical tools that are created with the help of your V-Self (your V-State Version). Each proxy is individual and very much your own creation, yet it is linked to all other proxies that have been and will ever be created. Once you have developed your proxy, it will help you to achieve V-State through a series of I-Self interactions (and Iterations).

Our E-State experiences will usually lead us to believe these interactions occur in time, through time and over time; however, our V-Self knows that all interactions occur in various states of potential and it is the conscious experience of each iteration that gives the illusion of time.

Our V-State invites us to decrease the number of iterations we consciously visit, before attaining V-State, whilst our E-State will focus on the time it takes to encounter each progression towards some distant experience. So, with each iteration of V-State, you have access to a huge repository of information that will help you create proxies of increasing value.

Therefore, when you work with vKRT, it is not simply a question of conducting a treatment for your client; within that treatment, the experience will be the clues and guidance to develop your treatment for the next iteration. When you Vvolve your treatment methodology through philosophy or proxy, in the process of all treatments, you will continually adapt and change the treatment from the foundation method to V-State treatments.

Now, the Viridian methodology of creating V-State proxies is a very specialised process so, for the sake of ease at this early stage of your KRT Journey and the One Therapy Practitioners' Experience, we shall look only at the basics of vKRT. These will serve as foundations and be built upon in KRT Mastery and the One Therapy Practitioner Programme.

For further information about One Therapy, please visit, www.one-therapy.com.

The very first proxy you are invited to construct will be a very simple object, such as crystal, a piece of wood or some form of metal, such as a ring, pendant, etc. As this is the first stage of your Viridian Vvolution, all you need do is choose a pre-existing object.

Once you have decided upon your object, have this with you during the calibration to your vKRT orientation. During the orientation process, your proxy will calibrate to V-State and act as the device that guides you further, through treatment and technique.

One very important aspect of working with the proxy in these early days is your ability to distinguish V-State from E-State (and vice versa). Therefore, during your training period, it is important to work with the tools, methods and techniques presented here. Whilst you will adapt your treatment style, this needs to happen in a gradual way, one that relies on V-State.

Having a firm foundation in the practices presented in this Home Experience will help you; whilst jumping ahead and doing your own thing, may make it harder to determine V from E at a later point of your Viridian Method.

This is intended not as a warning, but as an appreciation for how V-State works. When you have a clear and accurate knowledge of the I-Self foundations, these will act as a guide when you visualise new iterations of the V-State consciousness. We are so saturated in E-State from Everyday life that having a solid start is vital in knowing what to ignore and what to incorporate into your vKRT style.

The treatment method of vKRT is very similar to the other layers of KRT, except here you learn how to introduce proxies into the treatment to improve the scale and scope of results that are achieved for all within the treatment arena.

This introduction of proxies begins with your initial calibrated object and will then extend in proxies that work with the environment, experience and events of the treatment. These exist in your physical reality but depend more on how you define reality than what you do in the physical world.

For instance, in the physical world, you place your hands either side of your client's head and trigger the Arena tool; the important part of this process is defining the Box Arena. This does not exist in the physical world, but the physical world can flow through (be filtered by) that definition. So, your hands are not creating a box, but defining a place for the real world to voyage through V-State.

You will use your calibrated proxy to define greater degrees of detail within your treatments and, as you do this, you will free up consciousness to focus on V-State, rather than the steps of achieving V-State. When you master this, you will be able to access V-State instantaneously—the illusion of time will have no effect on your experience.

Creating Your RT (First Proxy)

This basic version of an RT Proxy was developed purely for the KRT practitioner and offers access to the range of vKRT treatments. The RT will help you experience a V-State environment where you can conduct powerful vKRT treatments.

(Note—As this device is not a full Viridian RT, it will only work within the context of vKRT, so if you wish to progress to a full Viridian treatment, you will need to work through the Introduction to the Viridian Method Home Experience; part of the One Therapy practitioner training.)

In many ways, the vKRT treatment experience encompasses all other forms of KRT treatment, whilst having its own, completely autonomous effect for your client. The difference in the vKRT treatment appears to be purely philosophical, affecting the approach we take to treatment rather than treatment methodology. However, the vKRT ethos completely changes the way the treatment is defined and how it works.

Where karmic, miasmatic and holographic treatments all have a connection to time, the Viridian perspective of KRT does not use any temporal references in relation to treatment. Here, time is seen as a symptom or side-effect that stems from the specific point you are treating. The RT proxy will help you to transcend your own experience of time (and your conscious reality within time), and create a direct treatment without temporal limitation.

For instance, let us imagine you experience flu-like symptoms in November one year and a chest infection in September the next year. In your experience through time, you catch a cold, recover, and then develop a chest infection ten months later. In the vKRT perspective, the cold and the chest infection are part of the same root cause and can be treated without consideration of time.

Your RT proxy is needed to create the V-State perspective of non-temporal treatment, with a basic RT being the absolute essential, whilst the Matrix RT and the portal RT will help you develop treatments further.

To create your initial RT, there is a two-step calibration process and accompanying audio companion for the orientation. The first calibration will enable you to create an RT, whilst the second can be used for additional RT development and encoding. Eventually, you will be able to create an RT without calibration. However, the audio companion will always be a guide for you, if needed.

Before you embark upon the calibration, you will need an object to encode as an RT; this is usually a crystal of some form (clear quartz works well), metal (such as a ring or pendant) or a piece of wood (many choose to sculpt a wand or ward to encode as an RT). Whatever you choose, the object needs to fit comfortably into your hand so that you can hold it for lengthy periods. Some use a pebble, others a wand-sized object.

You may simply choose an object in rough form—a pebble from the beach or piece of fallen wood; a pre-designed piece—jewellery, carved sculpture, etc.; or something that you actually create from scratch—if you enjoy crafts and feel ambitious, you might choose to work a piece of wood and inlay metal and crystals!

Once you have the item you want to encode, work with the audio companion to calibrate to the RT orientation.

When creating additional proxies, you can expand your source materials to include liquids, plants and other natural substances, such as dyes, natural fabrics and so on.

Using Your RT

When it comes to working with your RT devices, you conduct treatments through defining your therapeutic environment, followed by the results of the treatment and a few other palliative factors. The radical aspect of treatment to keep in mind with vKRT treatment is that all Viridian treatments are conducted on yourself.

The effects of treatment filter through to your client, but are always initiated from your perspective and are designed to shift your perspective (heal your holistic experience of the world), to where your client has transcended the issues that are causing them concern.

This can be challenging at first; usually bringing up various questions. However, the more you work with a V-State perspective and the greater the mastery you develop around the vKRT treatment environment, the easier and more natural treatments will become.

In simple terms, let us suppose a client is experiencing a psoric miasm dis-ease—they are in the reality of the psoric miasm. The very fact you are communicating with them means you also have an understanding (experience) of that psoric miasm. When you treat the miasm with vKRT, you do not just re-pattern the miasm, you modulate to a conscious experience (V-State) where that miasm never existed.

Once you have treated the miasm within yourself, the client either has to acknowledge your reality of the world, or simply disappear from it. Sometimes, clients do just stop visiting, but if they do come back for further treatments, they will have no choice but to align with your Viridia (V-State Reality).

To treat yourself in the therapy environment, you use your RT to transition you into V-State and then identify the point of connection between you and your client. The RT will also identify every instance of the connecting factors between you and your client, as well as between you and everybody you have ever met/will meet.

When you initiate the treatment through the RT, the V-State experience will change those patterns/connections in such a way that you will have no knowledge of them any more. As the patterns and connections change, there is a cascading effect that completely shifts your perspective of the universe.

In this way, you are treating your reality to transcend that reality, using the dis-ease and challenges your clients present to heal yourself and to heal them as a consequence. To the E-State perspective, this will all seem very wild and wonderful; however, as soon as you step into V-State, the complexity of infinite reality and possibility becomes completely tangible in its simplicity.

- As with all treatments, create a connection to your client. Then, with your RT in hand, use the following method to define and conduct a full vKRT treatment.
- Concentrate on the RT in your hand and run your tongue along the back and forth of your top, front teeth. Internally state that you want to connect to your RT.
- Run your tongue along your teeth again and request your connection to your client be scanned, defined and monitored.
- Now continue by triggering the *vPrimer*.
- After a few minutes, you should begin to feel a really good connection with your client.
- State internally that you want to "Treat all karmic, miasmatic, holographic or E-connections that link you with your client."
- Ask the RT to notice any contractive reactions to the treatment and to treat these.
- Run your tongue back and forth, along your teeth one more time.
- Start to move the experience of their auric field through the box, using your hands to decipher the flows/bounce.
- As you locate different dynamics, distortions and disruptions, constantly ask yourself "What is this?", "How is this affecting me?", "Where is it from?", and so on. Be aware of any synaesthetic response you attain and use these responses as a *way into* the regression experience (story).
- Once you have exhausted the experience of each event, run your tongue across your teeth and use the v*Clearing* until the event is diminished.
- Towards the end of the treatment, ask the RT to seal and soothe the treatment in this new reality.
- Ask if there are any other aspects of this reality that need to be treated and enable this to take place, if necessary.
- Thank the RT for the treatment.
- Bring your client fully back into the room.

Defining a Treatment Environment and Experience

Beyond the basic treatment, you can bring further RT devices into the treatment session to define both the experience and the environment. These add enormous benefit to the treatment because the more you define a treatment through environment and experience, the more focused and targeted the results will be.

This is not just a question of mapping out the space and experience during a single treatment but also beyond the individual treatment session. You can define your therapy space, office, home and even your client's home to continue treating. In this way, any contractive experiences you encounter after the treatment will be negated.

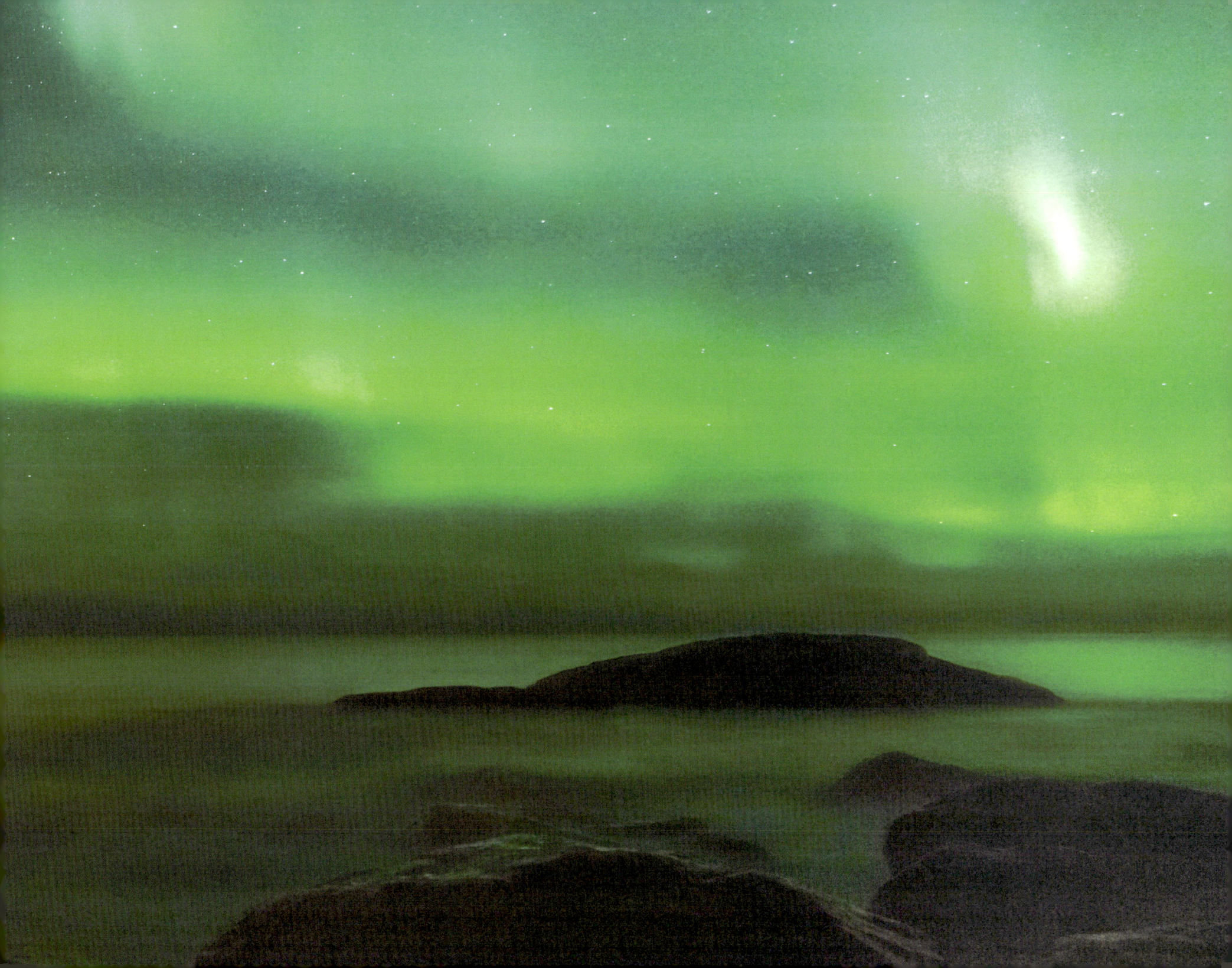

Furthermore, if a disconnection between you and your client occurs, the RT devices will endeavour to connect you both again.

Such an array of treatments for you to achieve with your RT devices takes extensive study and experience to master them all. However, this is the immense fun of vKRT! And it all begins with two variants of the RT—the Matrix RT and the Portal RT.

The Matrix RT defines a physical space and the environment of the treatment (meaning anything that is in or enters that physical space is encompassed by the treatment). A Matrix RT consists of an item for each corner (or boundary nexus) for the room. Usually, there are four items, one for each corner of a square room. Some rooms may need more crystals, pieces of metal, wood, etc.

Encode all the pieces intended for that Matrix RT by calibrating to the orientation, using the audio companion. Once this is complete, place each piece of the Matrix RT at a corner of the room, until it is completely defined by the nexus points. You will have given this matrix a unique name and can use this to identify the matrix during treatment sessions.

A Portal RT is an enclosed space of eight or twelve items, which focus the experience of treatment, rather than a specific area. Here, you and your client are situated within the completed portal, which focuses the treatment on the connection between you both (and any other factors that are defined with the portal).

So, whereas the matrix defines an environment, the portal defines a set of experiences, aims or results. This is very apparent when it comes to the ambient use of the Matrix RT to affect those entering a room, for instance. The portal would not affect those entering the physical space of the portal. However, you could trigger a specific treatment to be experienced by those already situated in the portal.

You can also use a portal to create a negative space or multi-tiered aspect to the treatment. So, a treatment may trigger through an RT Matrix, except in the area of a portal. Alternatively, a second treatment is conducted through a portal and targeted at a particular karmic/miasmatic event. Portals can be used to record treatments, that are then fed through a matrix and so on.

The portal is encoded much the same as the other RT variants, by calibrating to the RT orientation, using the audio companion. Here, however, you would ensure you have all eight or twelve items to be used in the portal with you at the time of calibration.

Increasing the Scope of vKRT Treatments

In the Viridian Method, a huge plethora of essences, treatments, resources and perspectives are curated for use in VM treatments. However, these add additional aspects to your vKRT treatments. You can, for instance, use one of the pre-defined essences for miasmatic clearing, whilst treatments for birth and death trauma also exist.

These are specifically for VM practitioners (VaMPs), yet there is a series of ways you can increase the scope of your treatments without VM training. You can record and playback entire treatment sessions, adapting these depending on the meta-level links between treatments—pinpointing common themes between say, five treatments, then treating these by theme, rather than in isolation.

If your treatment environment is not as you would ideally want it to be, you can define an area you have an affinity with (a forest, standing stones or other favourite location), through matrix or portal, then feed this through the matrix of your treatment room.

You can stack parallel treatments; comparing different outcomes without treating in the physical environment, before deciding upon the best treatment outcome from the comparison. You can even compile several treatments over many lifetimes to achieve results that we could not even hope to obtain in one lifetime.

The key to understanding the scope of your vKRT practice is getting to grips with how the RT devices work beyond time. Truly entering into the experience of consciousness without time and knowing how that translates to the role of the RT. This can be challenging for many because we have spent our lifetime addicted to time.

When we seek to transcend time, our conscious experience of life through time constantly draws us back into the addiction, so we have to be aware of how we experience our addiction to time and to make an informed decision about when we are functioning from the addiction and when we are not.

When you enter into V-State, the experience of time dissipates, and we experience all things through our expanded awareness, however E-State is tricky and can have us believing we are in V when actually, we are in E. The rule of thumb is, if you have any doubts that you are in V-State, you are not in V-State!

We can still visualise what non-time-specific experiences are, even when in E-State. To appreciate this, imagine an event through time. You encounter the event and pass through it.

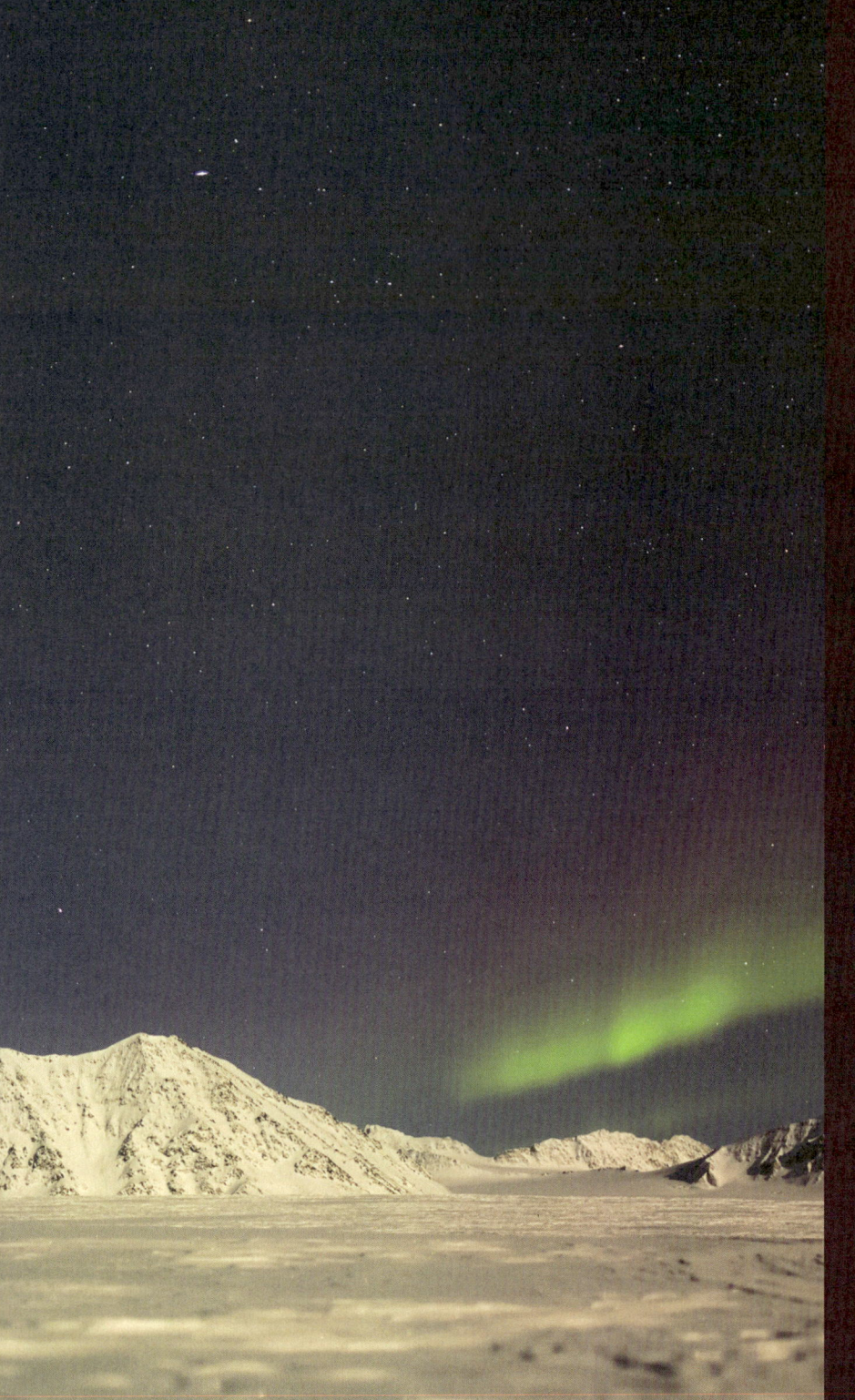

You remember the event in short-term memory and, if you remember the event frequently over a long period, the remembrance of the event is stored in long-term memory.

Beyond time, the event exists—it is not defined by time or even space. However, we can encode the experience of that event in various ways. Depending on what code we experience, we will experience a different conscious awareness of the event.

So, as an illustration, W is the event without any conscious experience of it; X is an actual conscious experience of the event; Y is a recent memory of the event; and Z is a distant memory of the event. When we consciously pay attention to this specific event, we will filter it through the code.

Beyond time, we are experiencing all events that possibly exist, with different codes; as soon as a code changes for a specific event, we have a different conscious experience of that event. Thus, in vKRT, you are treating the effects of an event by altering the code; altering a Z to a W, for example.

This is a highly simplistic view of the Viridian Methodology, intended as an interim whilst you are working towards V-State. However, it will serve you very well as a guide when you are struggling with time addiction. Also, keep in mind that your V-State self-knows exactly what codes are needed for all events, for you to experience V-State, so the more you transition into your V-Self, the easier V-State will be to master.

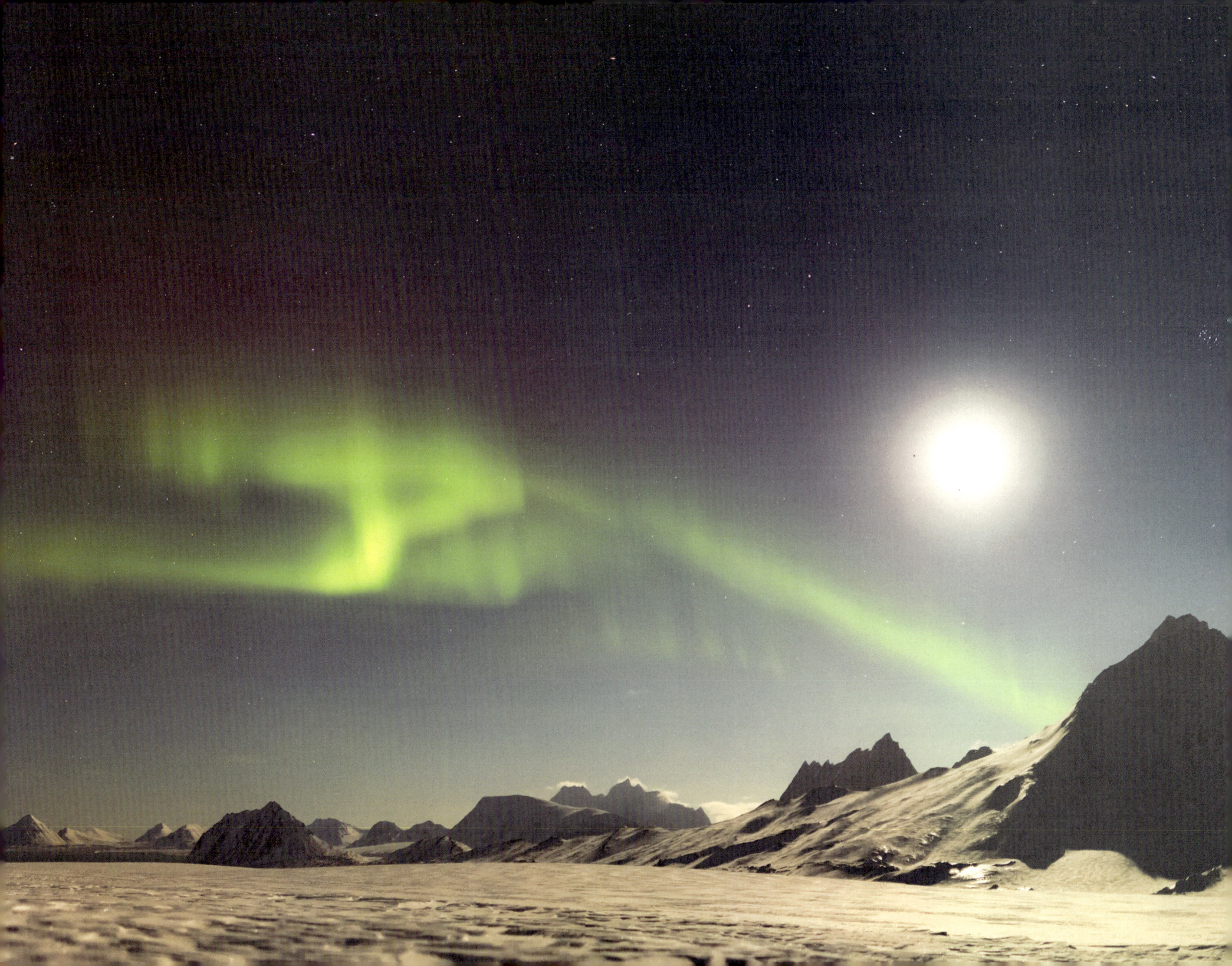

Practitioner Consultations and Feedback

Now that we have explored the different treatment methodologies of KRT and the philosophical wisdom behind each layer, it is time to investigate another cornerstone of our KRT professional practice—the consultation and feedback aspect of treatment.

In so many ways, these are an equally important part of your treatment style because you are essentially priming your client for treatment and then using imagery, metaphor and allegory to define their dis-ease (and how they can help the healing process initiated by treatment).

The consultation is the initial conversation you have with your client before the treatment takes place. This consists of three aspects; intent, hypnotic language, and memetic transfer. Then, we have the feedback from the treatment, which is where you illustrate and describe the different elements of the treatment experience, from your perspective.

During this portion of a treatment session, you are seeking to give the treatment context and meaning, as well as setting up a continued healing process for your client. This will ensure they continue to heal, long after the treatment has been completed.

The most important feature of these two elements is your professionalism throughout. Being aware of each statement and every word is so important—both consultation and feedback are carefully orchestrated pieces that weave through and beyond the treatment to form a fully-realised composition. A symphony of wellbeing and growth.

Many focus on the techniques and steps of treatment; conscientiously practising these to perfect their knowledge and style, whilst ignoring what happens before and after the actual treatment. The consultation is laying the foundations; the treatment is building the treatment; the feedback is cementing the treatment in place. Together, they expand the scope, greaten the depth, and lengthen the longevity of treatment.

As you enter into the consultation, your intent is to first define the boundaries (and thus, the focus) of the treatment. Here, you determine what your client wishes to focus upon, what results they want for the treatment and where they are currently. This is important because you cannot guide them to well-being if you do not know where they are starting from!

twelve

The focus of the treatment will influence the layer of treatment you work with, and the results are your guide to navigating the treatment—keeping these in mind throughout the actual treatment will help you maintain your bearings when in the complex terrain of the Box Arena.

During this consultation, you will also be instructing the client to remain open, to trust the processes of the treatment and to keep their focus on what they want to achieve. This will not only make the treatment more effective overall but will also help you to uncover the different aspects of their karma, miasma, holography and V-State to hone in on.

The use of hypnotic language is not intended to hypnotise your client but to relax them whilst keeping them focused on the end results they have defined. Mastering the hypnotic language and the principles behind this powerful means of communication involves in-depth study. Here, we will focus on a few basics that you can employ to improve the consultation process.

Hypnotic language can be based on a simple model of *suggestion and cover*. As you speak to your client, you have in your mind a suggestion you want them to comply with. This could be you want them to *relax and enjoy the experience*, or to *focus on their past traumas*, perhaps to *pay attention to your synaesthesia* and so on.

You then embed this suggestion within a complete sentence and cover it with peripheral words that give the sentence a different context.

For example a hypothetical... *It is so easy to just relax and enjoy the experience.*

A misdirect... *I often ask people to focus on their past traumas during the treatment.*

Or a completely obscured statement... *Sometimes, it is important to pay attention to your breathing and to keeping it calm as I work with the deep synaesthesia of the treatment.*

It is important to keep the statement fairly simple and always focus on what you want, rather than what you do not want. It is impossible to for us not to think about something that is mentioned, so if you ask somebody not to be frightened... they will hear *be frightened.*

When you present the hypnotic sentence to your client, you speak the cover words with your usual cadence (pitch, rhythm, accent, etc.) However, when you hit a suggestion word, you alter your cadence very slightly, maybe making the word a little deeper, speeding it up or using another accent. You can even distort the word slightly to make it sound unusual. Furthermore, you can construct suggestion phrases and keep these intact when covering them, even if the completed sentence does not make complete sense. so...

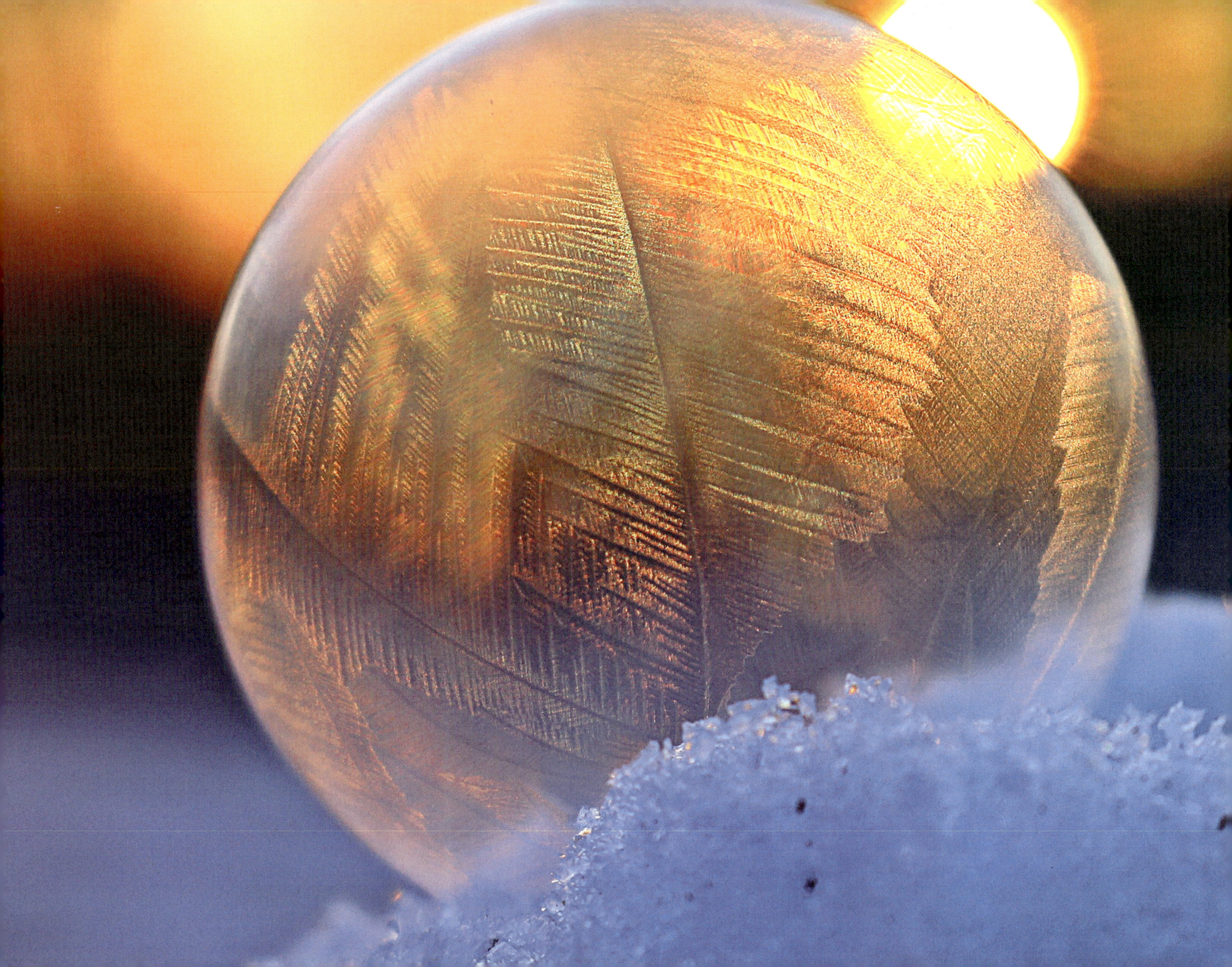

When I step outside my front door, and the more I walk...
you take a deep breath you relax deeper.

This may feel strange and, at first, you will be convinced your client will catch you in the hypnotic act, but if anything, they may be slightly confused. Remember that you cannot command a person to do what they do not want to do, so if they actively resist the hypnotic language patterns you offer, you cannot force them to get the most from the treatment or heal completely.

Beyond these embedded commands, you can also use a variety of other techniques to guide your client towards the best results from their treatment. *Pacing* uses descriptions through time to guide your client...

You pay attention to your breathing as you inhale deeply into your lower back and then very slowly exhale to a count of one, two, three, four, five, six and then just immerse yourself in a deep sense of wellbeing and relaxation.

Double binds offer the illusion of choice where there is no choice...

You could **deeply relax now** before we begin the treatment, or when you lay down on the table.

Then we have the convoluted and seemingly incomprehensible method of *extended quotes*, where you wrap a sentence up upon itself and have somebody else give the suggestion within a quote...

I regularly have clients tell me that their friends and family members comment to them after treatment how

"You look so healthy and are obviously getting immense benefit from your KRT treatments!"

Obviously, unless you undertake a full hypnosis qualification or already have done so, you are not a qualified hypnotherapist. These suggestions are the absolute basics of what is a vast body of study. Yet, practising and using these techniques will ease your client into getting the absolute most from treatments.

During a KRT treatment, we need our client to focus on the connection between them and their regressive trauma, be it karmic, miasmatic, holographic, etc. When they pinpoint this link, we will appreciate how that link reflects upon us and can treat that link through the desired treatment method.

In addition to hypnotic language patterns, we also focus on memes to develop new layers of treatment benefits for our clients during the consultation and feedback stages of the session. Memes are a form of autonomous entity that gain self-definition through transmission from person to person via the filters that create consciousness.

The memes that we encounter on a daily basis include songs, advertising slogans, fashion trends, spiritual and social beliefs, plus any form of communication that can be mimicked by other people.

It is this process of imitation that gives the meme its name, for *meme* comes from the Greek *mimos* —to mimic. Memes can, therefore, be regarded as replicators that define energy in a specific way and then communicate said definition so that others can replicate the results obtained by the definition.

Each time a meme is transmitted from one person to another, it gains additional dimensions of definition that basically create the information that the meme consists of. The meme is, thus, not force contained within a definition; it is the force of definition.

Memes are passed through consciousness at different layers of value in the parameters of space-time and, depending on the value layer, they will be processed differently. A consciousness may choose to connect to a meme and pass it on to short-term memory or it may choose to reject a meme.

Memes that are passed into short-term memory frequently enough will *stick* on a long-term basis, hence earning the title, *sticky meme*. A meme that is frequently rejected will eventually stop being transmitted altogether and simply cease to be in current space-time.

The exact processes behind meme transmission are quantified into a set of spheres—social spheres that determine what type of meme is transmitted and how this is interpreted by the recipient. In KRT terms, we define these layers as spheres of belief, as this provides us with a degree of multidimensionality, rather than linear progression of value layers.

When we apply these spheres of belief to our previous exploration of karma,

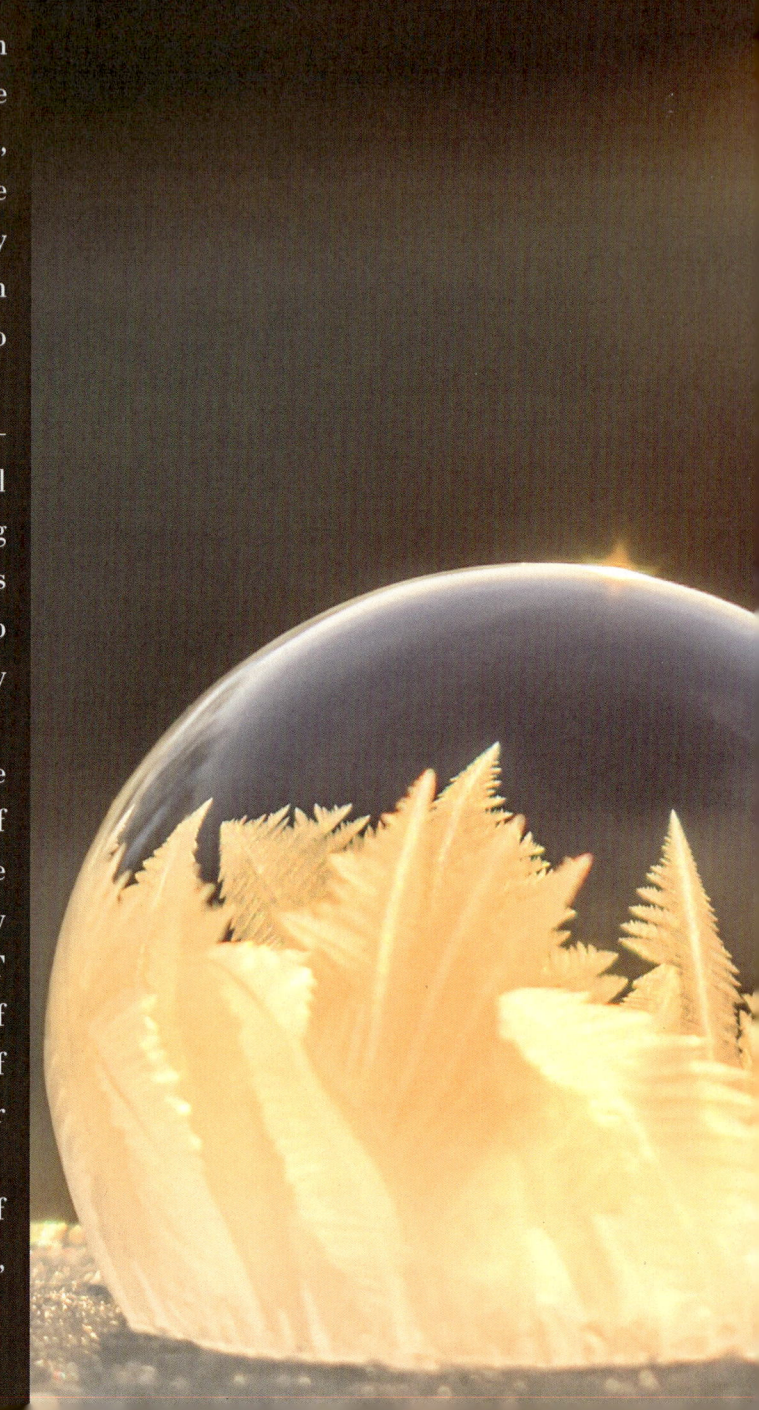

we realise that wherever the client is within the context of the six realms, will have a bearing on what they take from each meme. A client in the Titan realm will often react angrily to certain memes, whilst Hungry Ghosts will become more and more desperate for resolution.

The purpose of the memes in this context and from your professional perspective is to lead clients into the Human realm and then treat the journey they take—gaining an understanding of the path and learning how to re-pattern the path. By using memes to walk from one realm to another with your client, you will unlock the patterns they are working from, and prepare them for treatment.

If they are, even temporarily, in the Human realm for treatment, you will effect the greatest results from the session, so study, practise, and master your ability for memetic transfer.

Once you have established the various cornerstones, the treatment will take place, and you will gather various degrees of feedback to feed back at the end of the treatment. When it comes to this feedback, you are seeking to offer specific, definite, and targeting points your client can work with. These are both inspirational, contextual and deeply relevant to them (and their situation).

During this stage it is important not to present your client with vague and random thoughts—remain firmly on the results and goals of the treatment and filter your feedback to embody these. By giving the feedback a powerful and pinpointed message, you are consistently reminding your client of their accountability in the healing process.

Again, during the feedback process, focusing on hypnotic language and memetic transfer will keep the feedback honed on results. Here, however, you are reaffirming the results in relation to the experiences you had in the treatment session. If you have prepared your client for treatment, they will have identified a huge array of symbolism, imagery and solutions for themselves.

I would recommend that when you offer feedback, you start by explaining to the client what you experienced from the treatment, before asking them what they saw, heard, felt, etc. This is important, as the client may think you are simply repeating what they have told you if they relate their feedback first.

When you initiate the feedback process, they will be utterly amazed at how their experiences reflect what you discovered during the session. You can then link back your experiences with theirs and make concrete any natural links that have arisen.

This process of offering treatment feedback, obtaining the client's feedback and then tying the two together is a very potent way of sealing the treatment as one of real value. When both you and your client have been exploring the same areas of karma, miasma, etc., they will be even more determined to manifest results for themselves, and for you.

So, developing links, shared references, and clear connection between your experiences and theirs is an important aspect of sealing and reconciling the session into a complete package. The neat little bundle of consultation, treatment, and shared feedback will feel congruous and integrated, thus presenting both you and your client with a well-rounded experience.

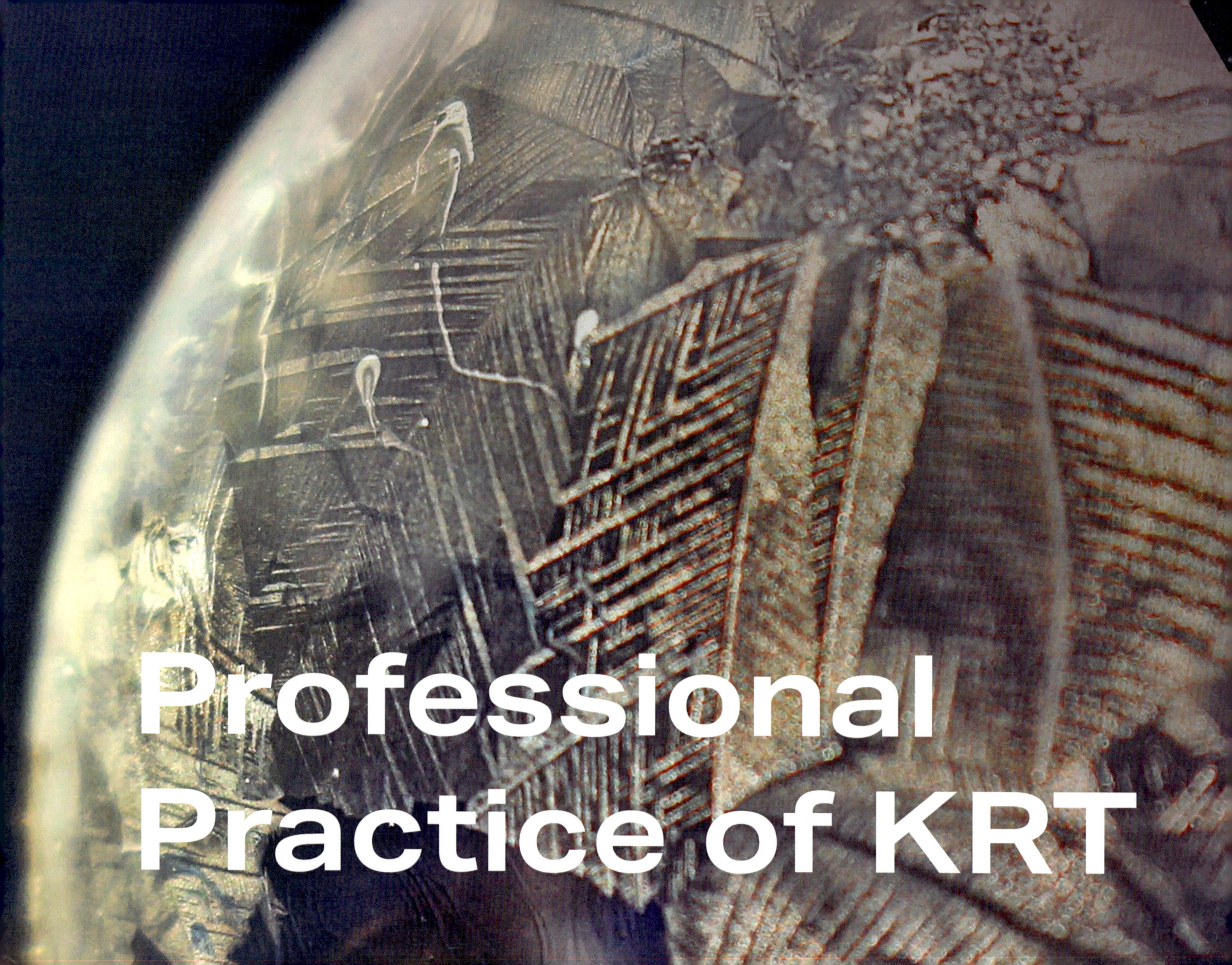

Professional Practice of KRT

thirteen

As you develop, refine, and perfect your one-to-one treatment sessions with clients, you are creating a valuable and effective way of making the lives of others and yourself better.

The transformative impact that you have on your client's experience of their world is at the core of KRT as a therapy.

In many ways, you are of service to your clients; seeking to be the catalyst in their attainment of a richer, more beneficial life. Yet, it is so easy to become lost in the words and platitudes, especially when it comes to a vibrational, energy-driven therapy such as KRT.

Therefore, it becomes exceptionally important to remain focused on the core benefits and definitive goals of a client's journey as you help navigate them along their treatment path. It is also equally important that you have this same clarity about your own healing path—in the range of results, the depth of impact, and the longevity of effects from every treatment.

For this purpose, having a master plan is essential to determine why you are serving others, what you are doing with consistency to help them, and how you are achieving all of this in a way that also benefits you. If you are just expending time and effort to give people a quick-fix or an ego-massage, you are not really helping them—and you are not living your legacy.

Insights such as these form the very heart of your professional practice. Your KRT business is not about making loads of money—it is the business of effectively serving others, making a better world and creating a solid legacy for yourself.

Your professional business does need to make enough money to support you, to keep the business going and to offer you a lifestyle with which you are truly happy. However, this is not the standard in most Reiki, energy or vibrational therapy practices.

When a practitioner has many issues around money they fail to charge an appropriate amount for their service. As a consequence, their business will usually fail. You would not expect to live very long without water to drink; businesses cannot survive very long without the money they need to thrive.

Yet, this is just one simple aspect of running a successful business. You not only need to offer top quality, professional treatments but also be able to communicate how transcendent the results are. You need to convince others of the benefits and you need to account for the relationship between results, income, and client satisfaction. Once you have done this, you can continue to develop a strategy that effectively creates your legacy.

Your business is your legacy—or at least an important part of it. And whereas many therapists offer treatments and never have any way of ascertaining the effectiveness of those treatments over time, your business is a very clear indication of how beneficial and valuable your service is to others.

When a therapist continually offers treatments to others without having a method of proving the effectiveness of treatments through the business, they are literally pleasuring

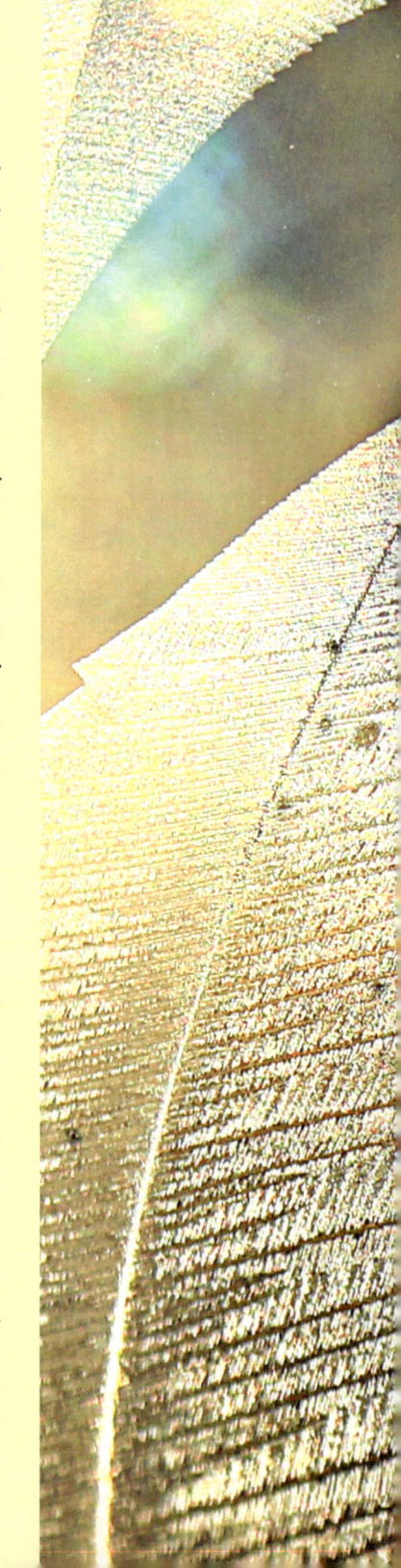

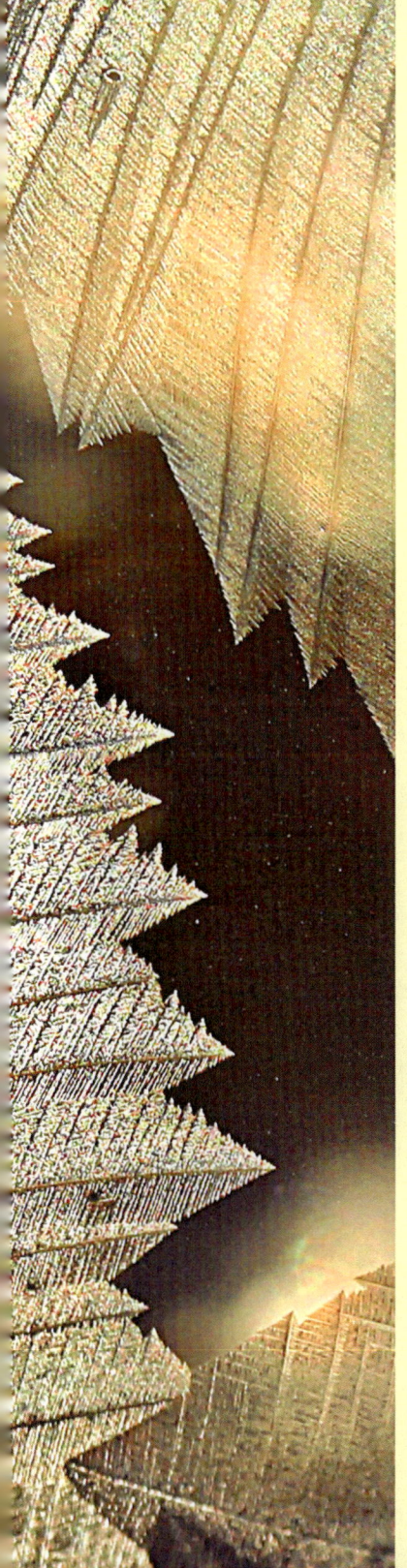

themselves. Going through professional life, safe in the knowledge that you are serving others but without actually serving others in a clear and defined way is ego-driven behaviour.

The most successful practitioners in our field are successful neither through pondering how good they are because they do not charge for their service nor because they have a big house and fast car. They are successful simply because they have regular, paying clients, who offer testimonials and referrals. Plus, even more so, because they have a legacy that will outshine their own lifetime.

Professional practice is proven through qualification, effective and definable business, and a powerful legacy. There is nothing wrong with offering treatments to friends and family, but we must differentiate between professional practice and helping others in one's own free time.

Of course, this dialogue all comes down to your own needs. If you seek to help others as an interest or hobby, then this is a rewarding and satisfying way to invest your time. If you are seeking to treat people professionally, then you must hold yourself accountable to the benchmarks of professional-level service, business, and legacy.

I truly admire people who give their time in service to others and the world. It is a noble and profound effort in which we all need to partake. I have absolutely no issue with people making a sustained and appropriate income from the business of their professional practice. What I do find very challenging are those therapists who set up businesses and then behave very snootily about others who are supporting themselves through their business.

If you want to work professionally, you will need to be professional. Firstly, through achieving your qualification, then by setting up and running an effective business and, lastly, through having a robust and ongoing plan for legacy. If you are not building a legacy that embraces some higher, benevolent and lasting results, then your business has no guiding principle to adhere to or strive for.

And so, we come to appreciate that our own legacy is at the heart of our business; for our legacy is the heritage of others—what they will inherit from us. And so, we see the connection between those who installed within us what we were born into, what we create and grow to offer others and those who will come after our own deaths—those who will continue our legacy onwards through time, and beyond it.

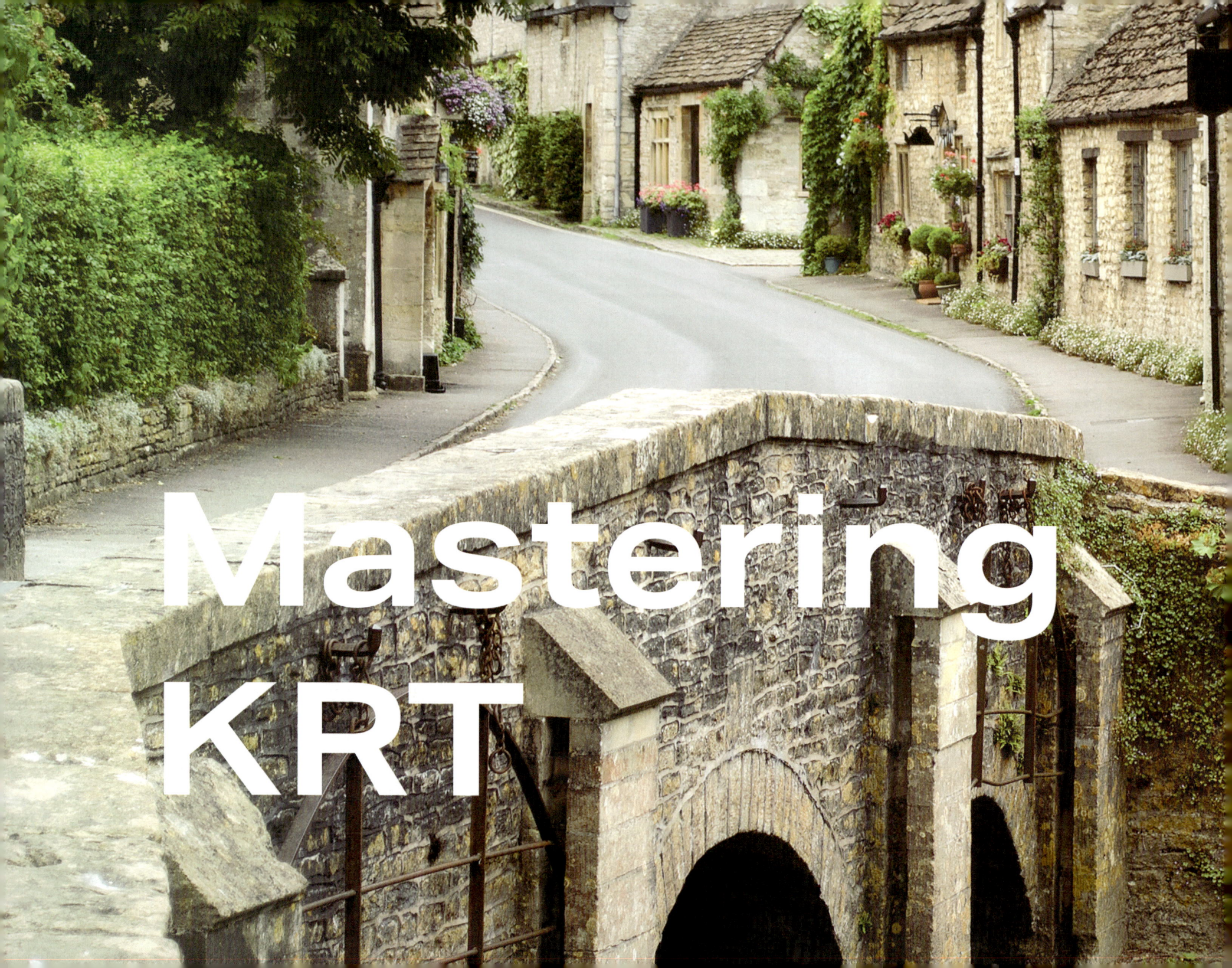

Mastering
KRT

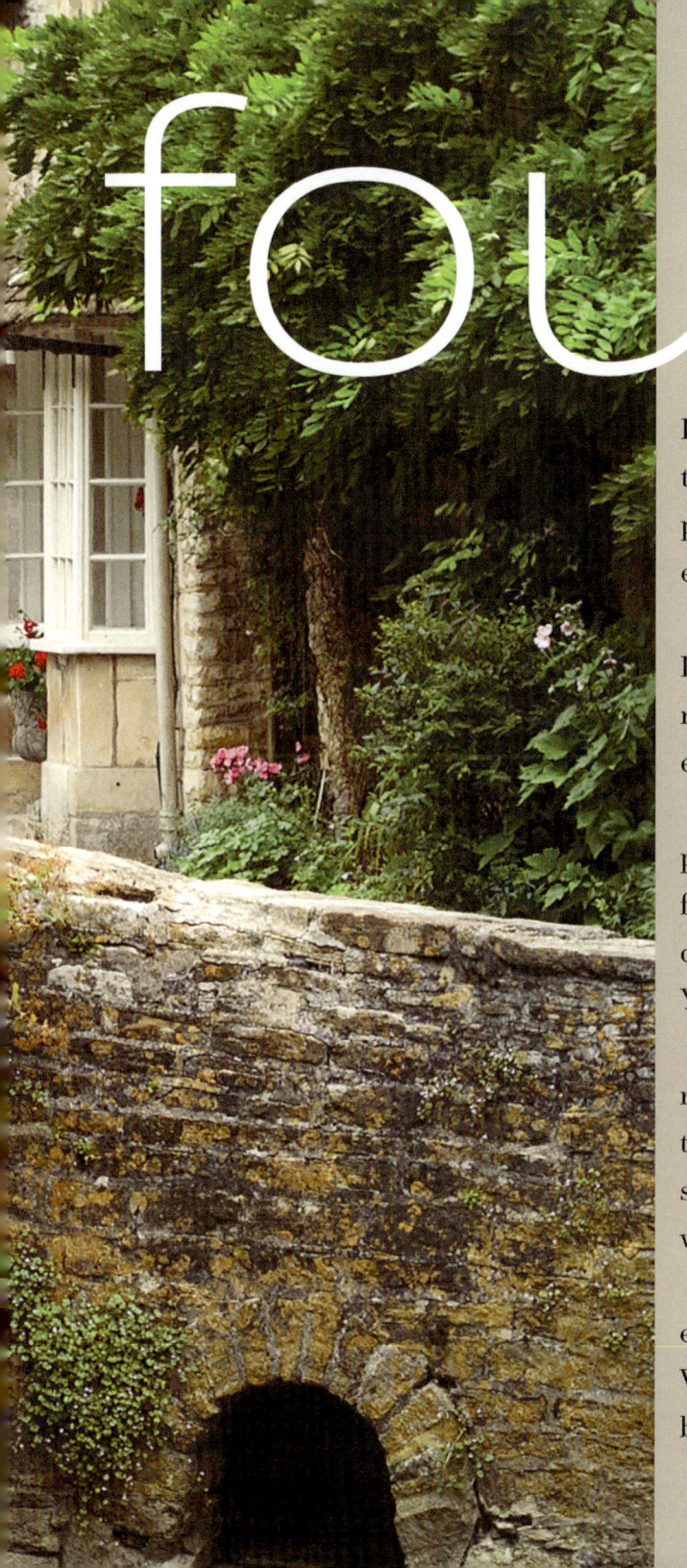

fourteen

Karmic Regression Therapy was created over time, and yet, through time it has come to transcend the very thing from which it was originated. Whilst the relatively simply practice and range of tools has changed slightly, the core ethos behind KRT has evolved from a simple philosophy to a vast, multifaceted, and trans-temporal method.

This can mean that there are three stages to the practice and mastery of KRT. First, the simple step of learning the tools and how to use them. Next, the more challenging perspective of intuitive reading, synaesthesia interpretation and explaining them to your clients in a coherent way.

Finally, we have the complex progression of the foundational philosophy that progresses from the concept of karma to miasma, birth and death holography, and finally to the Viridian perspective. All these combined and condensed into an intensive course will present you with a professional degree of understanding for your craft. Yet, to truly master the art of KRT at a practitioner level requires additional study.

The first and most important aspect of this study is to continue your practice, regularly, constantly, and congruently. Just as the origination process occurred over time, your practitionership can be honed and developed over a series of treatment sessions. The more you conduct these, the greater your understanding and experience will become.

Beyond this ongoing mastery of your practitionership, we also have the other elements of One Therapy practitioner, from vReiki and Celtic Reiki to PsyQ and the Viridian Method. These will not only offer contrast and nuance to your KRT practice but also develop your understanding of vKRT, professional and business knowledge,

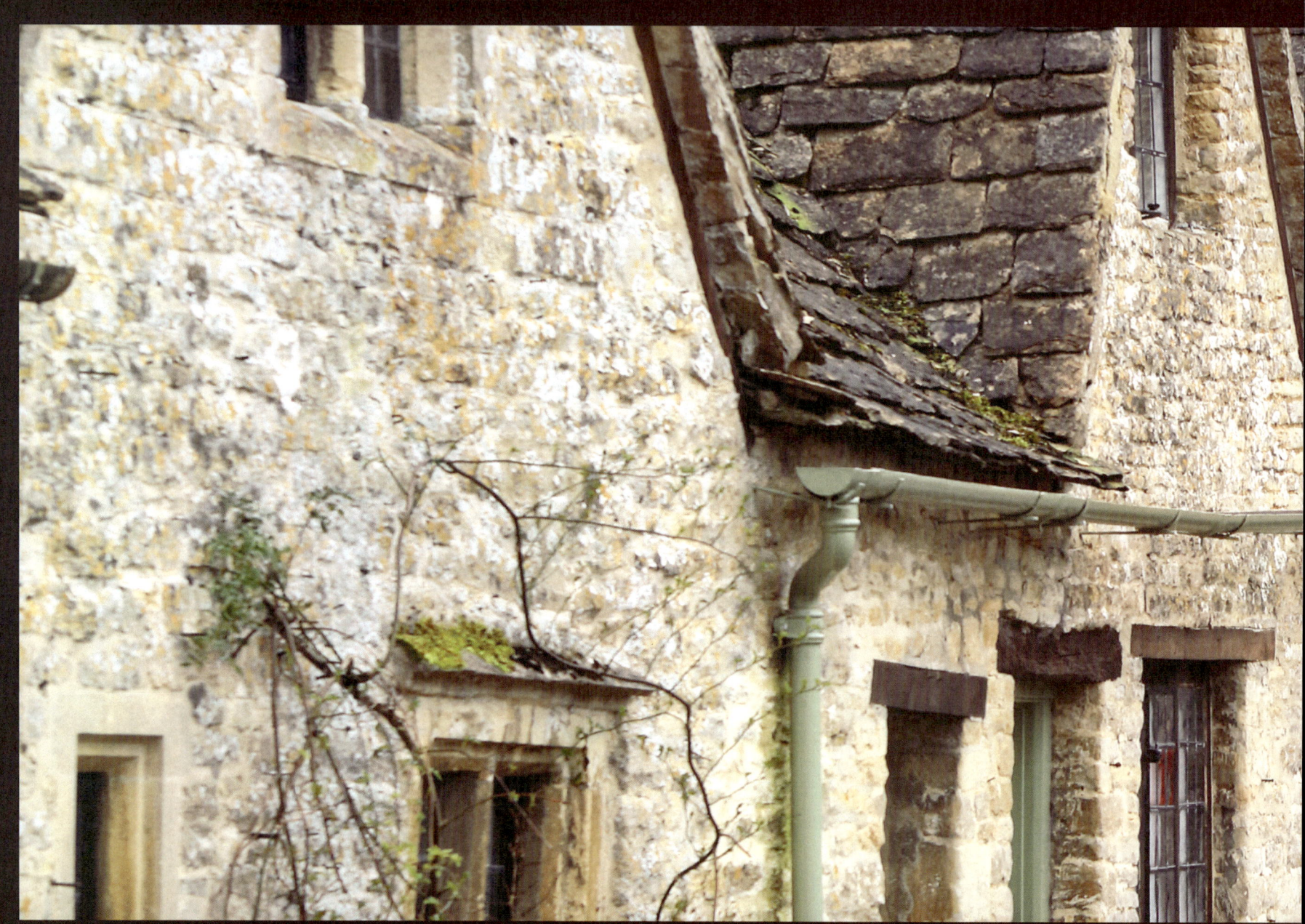

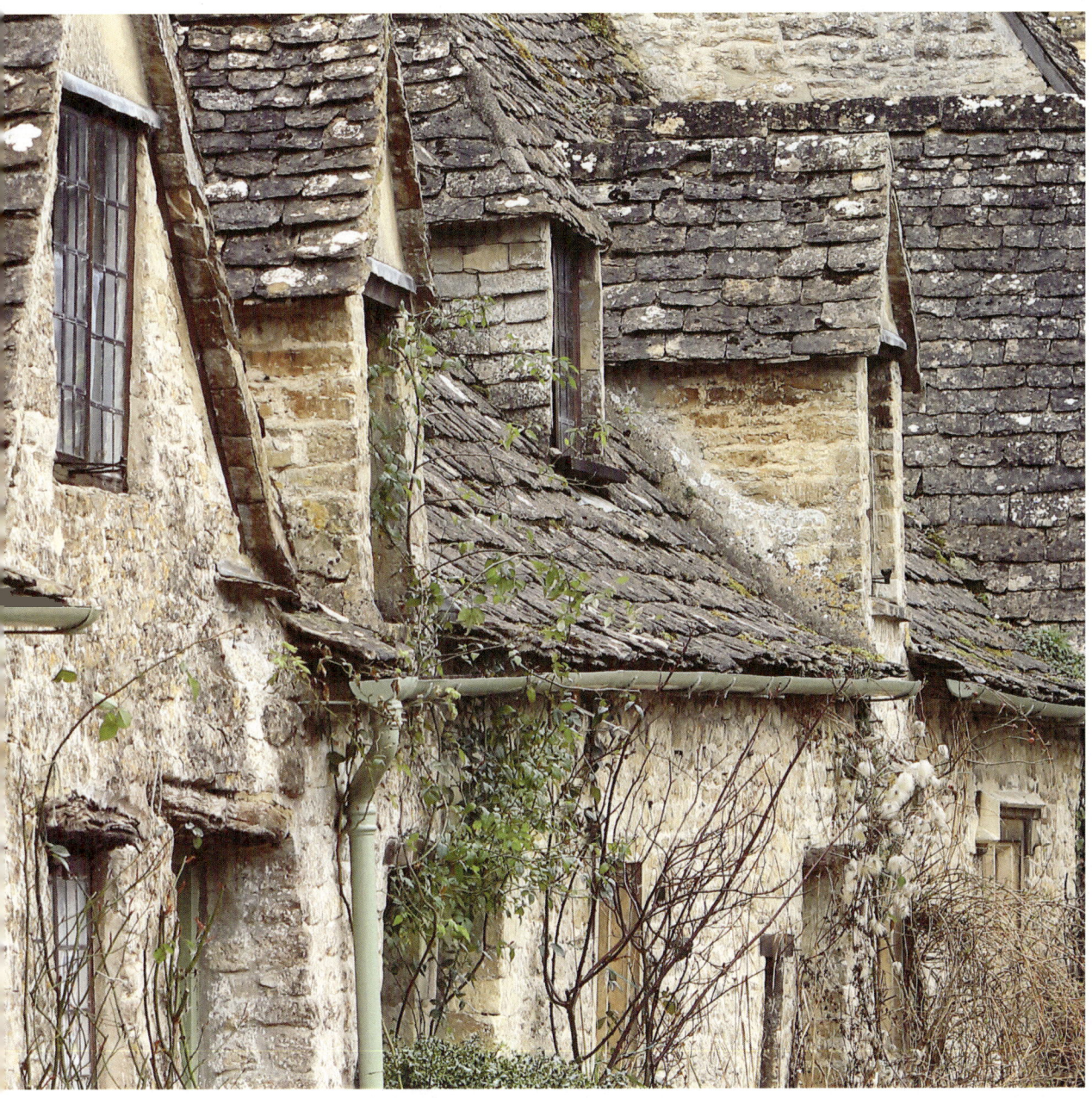

as well as increase your intuitive and sensory abilities.

Beyond One Therapy practitioner, the mastery of KRT and how you can progress your treatment of others to the teaching and mentoring of students will expand your knowledge of KRT in major ways.

Through all this, an important feature of KRT to keep in mind is that your journey remains the focus of your learning. As you encounter, appreciate, and transcend your own regression states, you will evolve as a person.

This evolution as person and therapist will underpin all that is to come. Striving towards your own healing and repatterning of karma, miasm, holographic well-being and your Viridia, will act as a constant guide; a map of the way forward and a record of all that you have done.

More than this, your legacy will exist beyond time... beyond the realms of karma and vibrational trauma of miasmatic heritage. Your legacy will create value in your birth and your death, whilst being a unique thread of the Universal Constant. This is the power of KRT and the wonder of all you are, in time and beyond time...

one

therapy home experience

www.one-therapy.com

Discover the extraordinary perspective in One Therapy—five life-changing forms of therapy in ONE.

Through the experiential journey of human connection, space, time, force and mind, you will know how to unlock the secrets that drive us all in the quest for oneness.

Empower yourself, create a professional approach to your therapy and transform the lives of others...

Lightning Source UK Ltd.
Milton Keynes UK
UKRC011251160721
387268UK00002B/12